extra lean

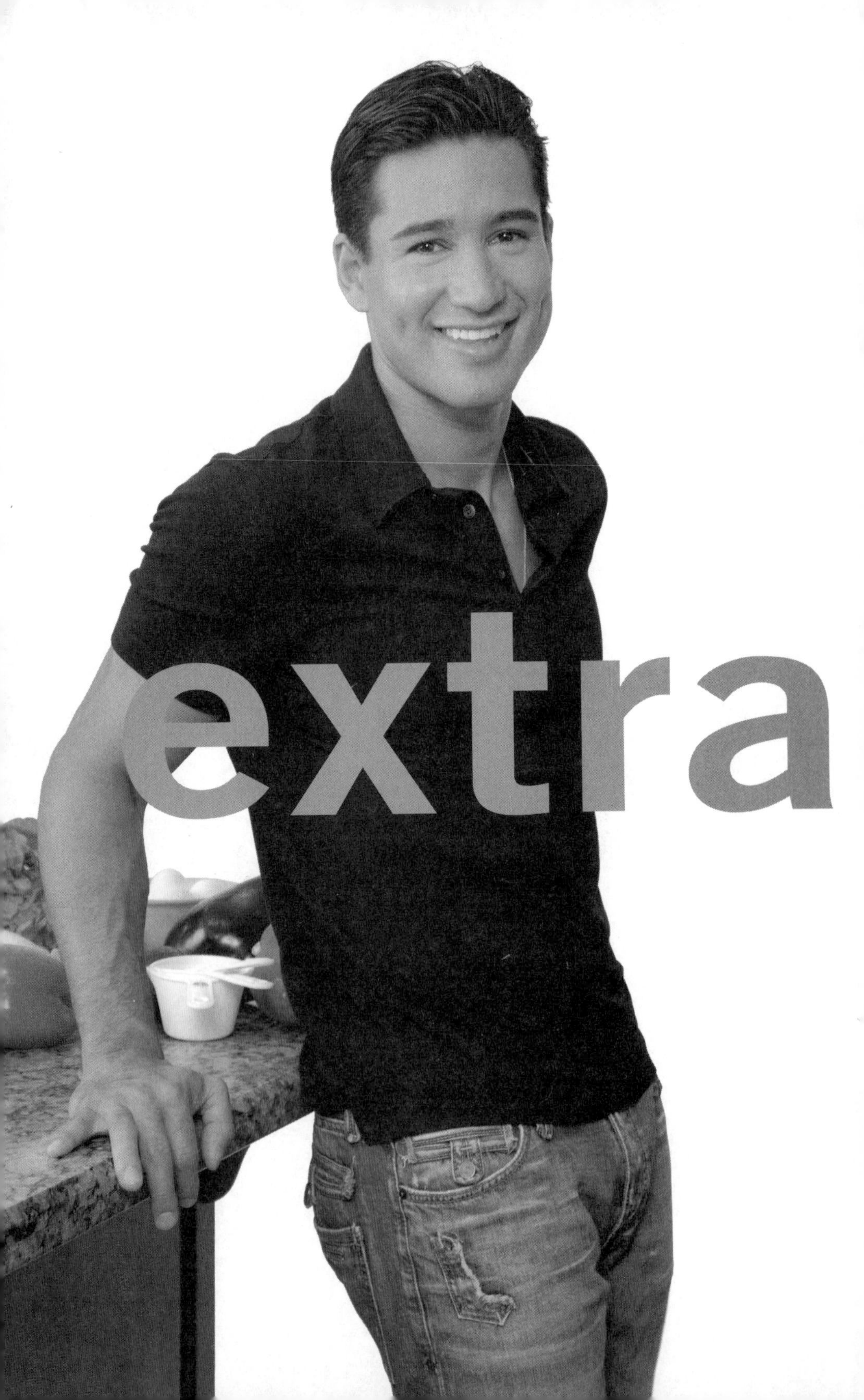
extra

MARIO LOPEZ

with JIMMY PEÑA

lean

THE FAT-BURNING PLAN THAT CHANGES THE WAY YOU EAT FOR LIFE

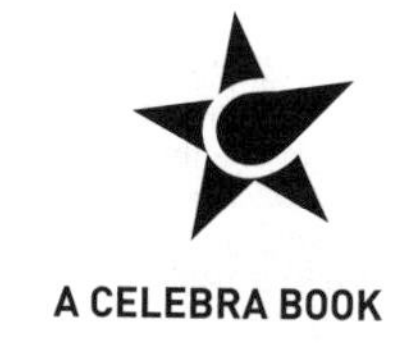

A CELEBRA BOOK

CELEBRA
Published by New American Library, a division of
Penguin Group (USA) Inc., 375 Hudson Street,
New York, New York 10014, USA
Penguin Group (Canada), 90 Eglinton Avenue East, Suite 700, Toronto,
Ontario M4P 2Y3, Canada (a division of Pearson Penguin Canada Inc.)
Penguin Books Ltd., 80 Strand, London WC2R 0RL, England
Penguin Ireland, 25 St. Stephen's Green, Dublin 2,
Ireland (a division of Penguin Books Ltd.)
Penguin Group (Australia), 250 Camberwell Road, Camberwell, Victoria 3124,
Australia (a division of Pearson Australia Group Pty. Ltd.)
Penguin Books India Pvt. Ltd., 11 Community Centre, Panchsheel Park,
New Delhi - 110 017, India
Penguin Group (NZ), 67 Apollo Drive, Rosedale, North Shore 0632,
New Zealand (a division of Pearson New Zealand Ltd.)
Penguin Books (South Africa) (Pty.) Ltd., 24 Sturdee Avenue,
Rosebank, Johannesburg 2196, South Africa

Penguin Books Ltd., Registered Offices:
80 Strand, London WC2R 0RL, England

Published by Celebra, a division of Penguin Group (USA) Inc. Previously published in a Celebra hardcover edition.

First Celebra Trade Paperback Printing, May 2011
10 9 8 7 6 5 4 3 2 1

Photography: Michael Darter
Food styling: Food Crew—Jeff Parker and Lisa Barnet
Grocery lists courtesy of Celsius® pre-exercise supplement drink—Your Ultimate Fitness Partner™

CELEBRA and logo are trademarks of Penguin Group (USA) Inc.

Celebra trade paperback ISBN: 978-0-451-23306-6

The Library of Congress has catalogued the hardcover edition of this title as follows:

Lopez, Mario, 1973–.
Extra lean: the fat-burning plan that changes the way you eat for life/Mario Lopez, with Jimmy Peña.
p. cm.
ISBN 978-0-451-23016-4
1. Weight loss. 2. Nutrition. 3. Energy metabolism.
I. Peña, Jimmy. II. Title.
RM222.2.L576 2010
613.2'5—dc22 2009051306
[B]

Set in Din
Designed by Pauline Neuwirth

Printed in the United States of America

PUBLISHER'S NOTE
The recipes contained in this book are to be followed exactly as written. The publisher is not responsible for your specific health or allergy needs that may require medical supervision. The publisher is not responsible for any adverse reactions to the recipes contained in this book.

While the author has made every effort to provide accurate telephone numbers and Internet addresses at the time of publication, neither the publisher nor the author assumes any responsibility for errors, or for changes that occur after publication. Further, publisher does not have any control over and does not assume any responsibility for author or third-party Web sites or their content.

>>>> To Mom.
In many ways, we're still at the dinner table together.
Bon appétit, salud, and I love you.

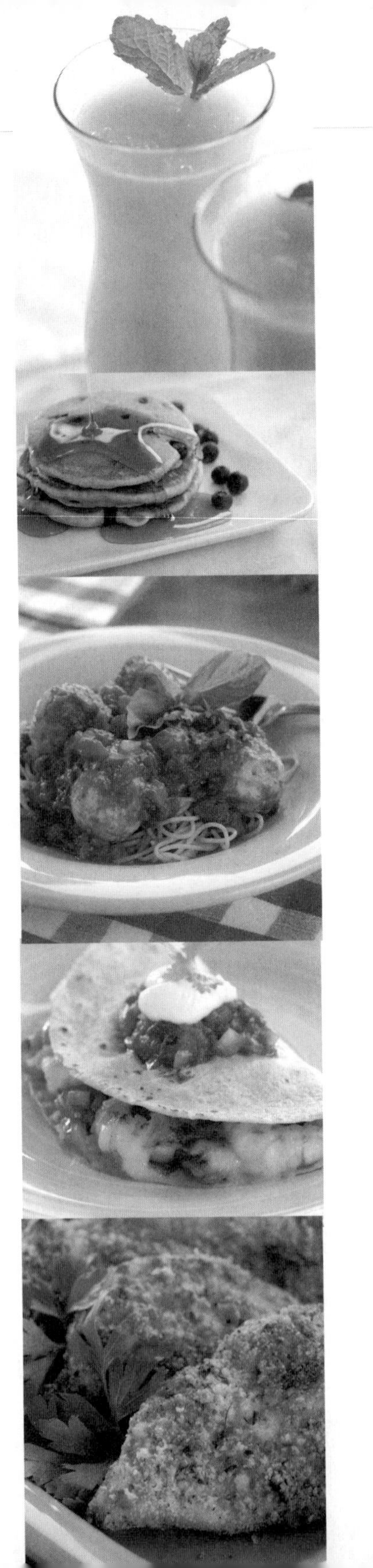

contents

extra lean

introduction: live extra lean

I LOVE FOOD. I love taking care of my body. I enjoy life to the fullest. I live extra lean.

When you live extra lean, the results are happiness and health. Through this proven plan, I'll teach you how to get the body you've always wanted and remove the guilt from eating the foods you love to enjoy.

Extra lean is the conditioning to make your body continuously burn fat, while enjoying food even more than ever. This approach teaches you to be smart when it comes to eating, so that you can truly appreciate what it means to live a fulfilling and energetic life. There are three key components in training your body to become extra lean. It is vital to follow these three simple rules to get your body to become a strong, efficient, and healthy fat-burning machine:

1. Balance your daily intake of carbs, protein, and fat
2. Practice proper portion control
3. Eat frequently throughout the day

Balancing your daily intake of carbs, protein, and fat is the first, and possibly most important, rule because it requires you to consume the basic nutrients necessary for your body to operate at its best. I'm all about balance, so I never cut any of these out of my meals or snacks. There are specific ratios of each nutrient that your body needs daily and, if you follow them properly, you can reach a level of efficiency that will allow you to eat whatever you want. This book simplifies the ratios of these nutrients so that you are able to know when you've reached your balance at every meal. It also provides knowledge about fundamental nutrition and an informative run-through on which types of carbs, proteins, and fats are healthiest and best for your body. Of course, focusing on whole, nonprocessed foods is a crucial component. Finally, this book introduces you to an array of incredible foods that are both delicious and great for your body.

Practicing proper portion control is knowing when to stop eating and understanding how much you should be eating. The key is to monitor your serving sizes. And the basic logic is that if there's less on your plate, you will eat less. First you have to redefine your "normal" serving size. Once you do, your mind and body will recondition themselves, allowing you to feel full and satisfied with the "right" amount of food. Also, learning your limits when it comes to the amount of food you eat will especially help in balancing all the types of foods you crave. Portion control is the most powerful tool in eliminating guilt.

Practicing proper portion control is knowing when to stop eating . . .

Eating frequently throughout the day allows you to better control your portions and speeds up your metabolism, making your body burn more of the unwanted fat and calories instead of storing them. As you practice this rule you may be feeling that eating more often is slowing down your weight loss, but it is actually speeding up your metabolism. Think of your metabolism as a furnace. In order to keep the fire burning, you have to constantly put something in there to maintain the heat. The same is true for your metabolism. You have to eat throughout the day in order for it to keep burning the fat. Doing so will help you lose weight more quickly and keep you feeling full and satisfied.

Following these three rules is all you need to maintain your weight and to burn fat daily. The reason being is that all three combined help you focus on what is most important when it comes to food and weight loss. This way of eating will jump-start a healthy lifestyle and in turn you'll have more freedom to eat whatever you want. I love food and that even includes a cheeseburger and fries from time to time. My entire life has been about living extra lean and that's allowed me to always enjoy food.

Eating frequently throughout the day allows you to better control your portions . . .

My life in the Lopez household always revolved around food. Cooking meals and eating right are how my mom and my sister showed me love and affection. Food was such a big part of our lives and we always tried to eat as a family. And despite my busy lifestyle and career and frequent traveling, I always look forward to and make time for meals, especially those with my mom and sister.

Growing up in Southern California, we always had an array of foods. Of course we had good Mexican food, which I'll admit wasn't always the healthiest, but I ate such controlled portions and so often that I just burned it all off. I ate constantly and, without even knowing it, I was eating in ways that were going to benefit me for a long time to come, not just physically but emotionally as well. As I've gotten older and become more involved in health and fitness, I've learned that my mom had it right all along. She always served me a variety of foods throughout the day, making sure I was constantly eating, no matter what I was pursuing.

Unfortunately, it's not this way for everyone. For far too many people, mealtime is a struggle. It's a time of uncertainty, of deciding what you can and can't eat and how large your portion sizes are allowed to be. Eating often triggers feelings of guilt, if the food isn't healthy, or feelings of being restricted, if it is healthy. But this isn't the way it should be, and that's why I'm writing this book. My approach to abundant health will get you to love food and achieve your desired body.

Thanks to my upbringing and following the three rules of eating the extra lean way, my body is now conditioned to burn fat at the most optimum level. It is second nature to me because I'm accustomed to consuming the proper amounts of carbs, fats, and proteins just by glancing at a meal. By sticking to my portion sizes, I'm satisfied at just the right amount of food and never feel too full or too hungry. My metabolism is at a constant state of efficiency because I eat frequently throughout the day.

The three rules allow my body to constantly burn fat. It is so incredibly liberating to eat whatever I want without guilt. Those who have yet to realize the benefits of maintaining an efficient body will constantly be at odds with maintaining their weight and enjoying food. I promise you that once you start following the three rules of living extra lean, you'll never feel bad about food again. When your body is in a state of living extra lean and has become a fat-burning machine, you can afford to splurge on days, weekends, and vacations with little to no effect on your weight and physique.

This book is armed with powerful tools that are backed by fitness expert and author, Jimmy Peña, and nutritionist, Dana Angelo White, MS, RD. With their help, I wrote this book to show you how to pick the right balance of wholesome, nutritious foods, and combine them to create great-tasting meals, with over forty original recipes. Because this plan introduces the right foods to detox your body and in the right amounts, you are creating the proper environment for successful weight loss. By the first fourteen days of completing the meal plan, you can expect to lose as much as fourteen pounds. You'll also learn how to measure the proper amounts of food you consume and regulate your body and mind to naturally adhere to portion control. Finally, I will give you a detailed breakdown of the specific times you should be eating and provide a logical method so that eating throughout the day will become second nature. These are the key factors of food that you need to balance in order to eat well over the long term with the right foods and the right amounts without sacrificing taste. This book also includes some helpful tips to maintain your new, lean body in your everyday life. From on-the-go options for those who don't have time to prepare a meal, restaurant survival tips, and frequently asked questions, this book is filled with effective resources that will keep you loving food, life, and your body.

After reading this book, I want you never to see food the same way again. I want you to view food in so many different ways. I want you to see food as a means to healthy living and a source for energy. I want you to see it as something you should enjoy. I want you to be in control and command so that you can experiment with different foods and enjoy a variety of meals. Food can be so many things to us, and it's only after you've made the decision to take control that food can be all those things to you.

The fact that you're reading this book is a testament to the notion that you want both happiness and health. You want to be able to enjoy food and life without obsessing over your weight and whether one night of indulging will have serious consequences the following day. If you'll just commit to learning about nutrition and following the three rules of living extra lean, you'll never be at the mercy of food again.

I'm thankful for my upbringing and for how my family treasured mealtime and taught me life principles about how to view food. Now I can help you along your journey toward success, abundant health, happy eating, and extra lean living.

I always knew Mom was smart.

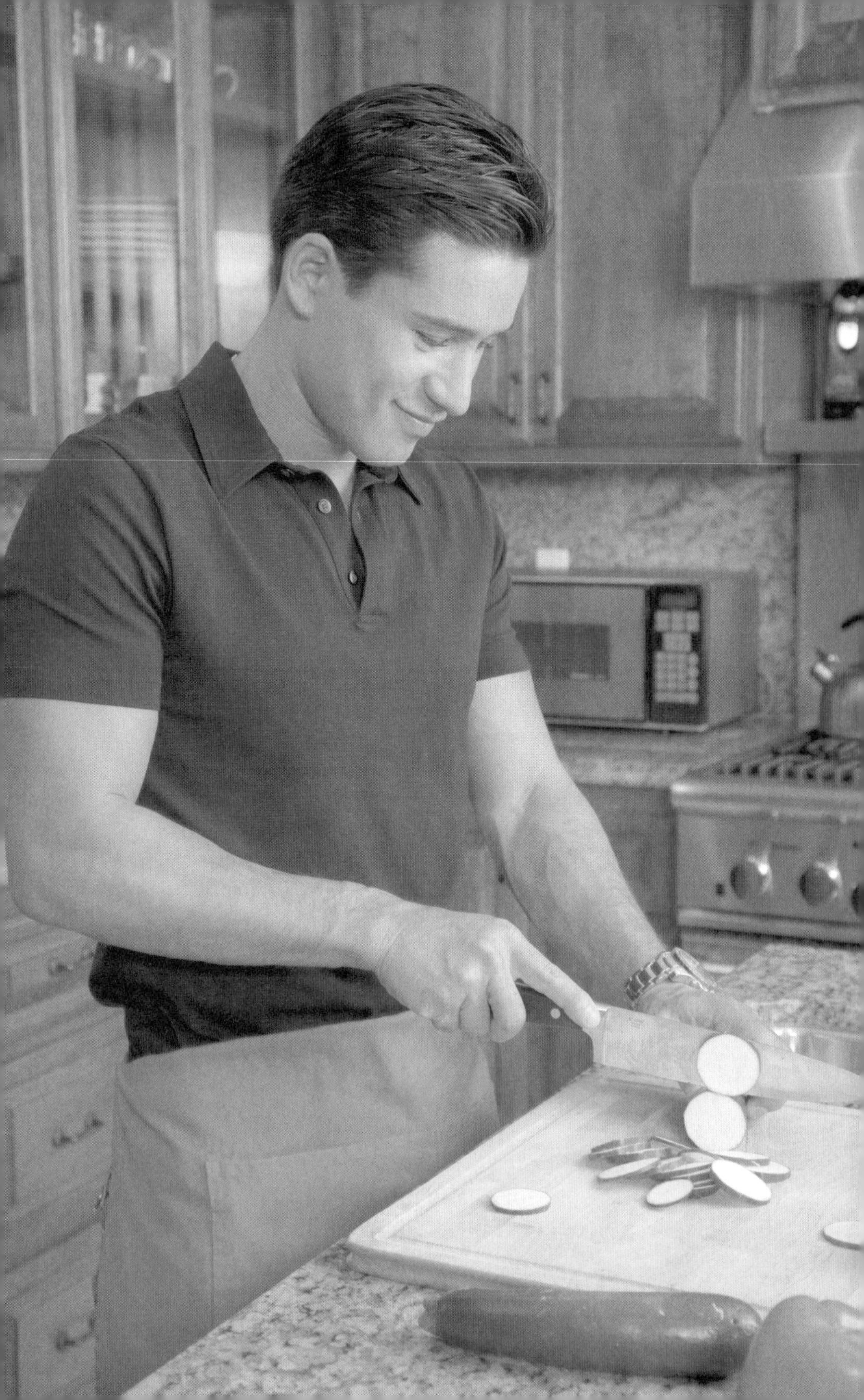

SECTION 1

the extra lean plan

TO CONDITION YOUR body to constantly burn fat and calories at the most optimum level, you need to follow daily the three simple steps:

1. Balance your daily intake of carbs, protein, and fat
2. Practice proper portion control
3. Eat frequently throughout the day

These steps are essential tools to identify optimal combinations of daily nutrients and learn transformative eating habits and invigorating mental conditioning. These are the only resources you will ever need to stay lean and enjoy food. This plan makes sure that you're nourished and energized, but only as much as you need to be so that you're not overeating.

You have my word that in the first fourteen days you can lose up to fourteen pounds, but this plan goes well beyond any weeklong or monthlong span. If you have a major weight-loss goal and follow the weekly meal plans in this book, you will reach your goal—and keep it. How you eat food is just as important as what you eat when it comes to weight loss. These three steps condition you to effectively approach food with the goal of both enjoying food and using food as a way to maintain a lean and healthy physique.

STEP 1.

balance your daily intake of carbs, protein, and fat

THERE ARE THREE basic macronutrients that the body needs to function properly: carbohydrates, protein, and fat. I wouldn't trust any diet plan that eliminates one or severely skimps on the other. The Extra Lean plan makes all of these nutrients work *for* you and not against you. Probably the most crucial of all the steps, balancing a combination of healthy carbs, protein, and fats throughout each day, ensures that you'll have plenty of energy to constantly burn fat and stay lean for life. To reach this state, you need to have the following total daily intake of each nutrient:

½ (more or less) of carbs

¼ (more or less) of protein

¼ (more or less) of fat

You may not always hit the exact amount for each nutrient, which is completely fine. The basic principle here is that you need to aim for those amounts daily to create a proper balance since all three enable the body to perform at its most optimum level. There is a higher amount of carbs because this macronutrient is the preferred fuel source of our cells; thus, creating an efficient environment of good carbs is the best way for long-lasting success. The daily intake of protein and fat, about one-fourth for each, is just the right amount to keep the body satisfied and to help curb cravings.

daily intake of carbohydrates

Carbohydrates are the body's preferred energy source, and your brain relies on them exclusively to function. If you keep your carbs very low, like many people do on low-carb diets, you can imagine how that may affect your performance. About half of your daily nutrient intake should come from carbohydrates; this is the perfect amount to give you plenty of energy and promote weight loss. Here's why: From a physiological standpoint, when there are inadequate amounts of carbs available in a meal or snack, the body doesn't have what it needs to work efficiently. It then must resort to releasing previously stored carbohydrates or battle to convert other macronutrients into carbs so they can then be used for energy. A half of daily intake of carbs allows your body to stay on track and rely on the proper energy sources to efficiently burn calories while keeping you satisfied.

Thus, it is a common misconception that carbs make you fat. When the right kinds are eaten in the proper amounts along with protein, carbs actually do the opposite. Notice I said the *right* kinds—the type of carbohydrates you choose are crucial to losing weight.

SOURCES OF healthy carbohydrates

- Fruit
- Vegetables
- Whole grains
- Legumes
- Nonfat yogurt/milk

Simple vs. Complex Carbs—Carbohydrates can be broken down into two main categories depending on how they're *broken down* by the body: simple and complex. Simple carbohydrates are quickly digested and burned for energy, and some are healthier than others. Healthy examples of simple carbs include fruit, milk and milk products like yogurt, as well as certain kinds of white bread. There are also some simple carbs in vegetables, which are also considered healthy. Sugar, candy, and soft drinks also fall into the simple carb category, but, as you probably know, are a lot less nutritious than fruit and dairy. Think about it—an apple has nutrients like vitamins and fiber along with those carbs, while something like candy or soda has only *empty* calories.

Complex carbohydrates take longer to digest and provide a more steady delivery of energy. These kinds of carbs typically contain good amounts of hunger-fighting fiber and various vitamins and minerals. Complex carbs are found in legumes (beans, peas, and lentils), starchy vegetables, and whole grain cereals and breads. Fruits and vegetables contain a combination of simple and complex carbs, and they also pack in a ton of vitamins and minerals relative to their low number of calories, which makes them perfect for getting in all of your vital nutrients while trying to lose weight. The goal is to eat a combination of healthy simple and complex carbohydrates from the foods that pack in the most nutrients.

When I'm deciding what to eat at a given meal, specifically where carbs are concerned, I always look for the big three: fruits, vegetables, and whole grains. If my carbohydrate of choice falls into one of those three categories, I know I'm good to go. Dairy is a good source of healthy carbohydrates, too, and it also provides good protein and fat. Carbs from sugar, candy, and soda, on the other hand? These are empty calories that I really try to steer clear of.

SOURCES OF whole **grains**

- Whole wheat bread, English muffins, and tortillas
- Brown rice
- Oatmeal
- Whole grain cereals
- Whole grain pastas

daily intake of protein

The main function of protein in the body is to build and maintain muscle to keep you lean and strong. Protein is also involved in numerous chemical reactions to regulate metabolism and keep cells healthy. Unlike carbs, which are all about energy production, protein is more about structure. Carbohydrates provide the energy needed to make sure muscle cells scoop up protein and (along with exercise) convert it into lean body mass (a.k.a., muscles). Protein is also digested differently from carbs; the structural pieces of protein take longer to digest, so they tend to keep you fuller for longer. About a quarter of your daily nutrient intake should come from protein, which allows the body to burn calories and body fat while you are active and at rest, maintain lean muscle, and avoid cravings.

Lean vs. Fatty Sources of Protein—When it comes to protein, the leaner the source, the better. Sure, heavily marbled cuts of meat have protein, but they also come loaded with high amounts of artery-clogging saturated fat, cholesterol, and extra calories. Stick to lean meats like chicken and turkey breast, pork tenderloin, and lean cuts of beef. Seafood is also lower in fat and calories yet packed with healthy protein. Eggs and dairy are good sources of protein too. There are also some great vegetarian sources of protein, like beans, legumes, and whole grains.

SOURCES OF lean **protein**

- Chicken breast
- Turkey breast
- Tofu
- Seafood: shrimp, cod, mahi mahi, tilapia
- Lean cuts of beef and pork

daily intake of fat

Fats are the third and final macronutrient, and just like carbs and protein, they play their own special role in the body. This nutrient's important functions include hormone production, nervous system function, shock absorption in joints, and temperature regulation. Like carbohydrates, fats are also burned for energy during different intensity levels of exercise.

Fat has gotten a bad reputation for causing weight gain, but the truth is that eating the right kinds of fat in the right amounts can actually help you lose weight more easily. As with protein, it takes your body longer to digest fat than carbohydrates. This keeps you feeling satisfied and gives you longer-lasting energy after a meal. But keep in mind that fats are a more concentrated source of calories—a gram of fat has more calories than a gram of carbs or protein, which means that portions need to stay in check.

"good fat" vs. "bad fat"

Fats probably have the worst reputation out of all the three macronutrients, but Dana has taught me to look at fat from a slightly different perspective. Those "bad" fats are either saturated fats or *trans* fats. Eating too much of these types can lead to high cholesterol, clogged arteries, and heart disease. (See the table below for a list of foods that contain saturated and *trans* fats.)

It's important to recognize that there are small amounts of saturated fats in healthy foods like milk, cheese, meats, and fish, but this doesn't make them "bad" foods, as they also contain healthy components like protein, calcium, vitamins, and heart-healthy fats. (In fact, fish is one of the best sources of fat as it contains high levels of Omega 3, a fatty acid that helps to reduce the risk of heart disease among many other health benefits.) It does mean, however, that you need to pick and choose where these foods should fit into your diet. You should seek all these good nutrients, but you should also moderate your intake of saturated fats and calories to keep your weight under control and your heart healthy. Trans fats, on the other hand, offer little or no healthful benefits and should be avoided as much as possible.

SATURATED FATS	TRANS FATS
Fatty meats	Commercially prepared baked goods like cookies, cakes, and pies
Cheese	Snack foods like chips and crackers
Butter	Some fried foods like doughnuts and certain brands of french fries
Lard	Some brands of peanut butter
Whole milk	Anything with "partially hydrogenated oils" on the label
Ice cream	
Palm kernel oil	
Coconut oil	
Cocoa butter	

Then there are the "good" fats, the ones that are unsaturated and help keep cholesterol low and the heart healthy. The two main types of unsaturated fats are monounsaturated fatty acids (MUFAs) and polyunsaturated fatty acids (PUFAs). Foods high in MUFAs include olive and canola oil, avocados, and peanut butter. PUFA-rich foods are salmon, safflower oil, walnuts, and sunflower seeds. It's also important to know that almost all foods that contain fat contain various combinations of these different kinds, not just one or the other.

Omega-3 fatty acids are PUFAs found in fish like salmon, tuna, sardines, and anchovies, as well as flaxseeds, walnuts, soybeans, and wheat germ. Omega-3 fats are especially important for growth and brain function, and they also help reduce the risk of heart disease and stroke by lowering cholesterol. Omega-6 fatty acids are PUFAs as well and are found in soy, meat, poultry, eggs, nuts, and seeds. A very interesting thing that I've learned is that the body cannot produce either of these special fats, the only way to get them is to fit them into your diet. Experts tend to agree that most people get more than enough omega-6s but fall short on the omega-3s, so it's best if you get a variety of both.

To make sure you're getting enough healthy fat, choose plant oils like olive and canola along with nuts, seeds, olives, avocado, fatty fish, eggs, and low-fat dairy products. It's funny—most people who spend a lot of time with me probably think I'm on a very low fat diet, but that's not the case at all. I love to cook with olive oil, snack on nuts and seeds, and eat salmon for dinner and eggs for breakfast, and all of these foods have decent amounts of fat, yet they're all healthy. What a trip!

other important nutrients

FIBER

Fiber is a super healthy type of complex carbohydrate. Found mostly in fruits, vegetables, legumes, and whole grains, fiber-rich foods also come packed with a ton of other healthy nutrients like B vitamins and antioxidants. Eating fiber-rich foods helps keep you energized and satisfied longer, so it's a good idea to spread your fiber intake evenly throughout the day.

There are two main types of fiber—soluble and insoluble—and each has its own unique health benefits. The soluble fiber in oats, barley, legumes, and citrus fruits helps to lower cholesterol and keep blood sugar levels stable (this helps you avoid drastic surges and dips in energy levels), while insoluble fiber is found in whole grains, nuts, seeds, and vegetables and helps with digestion. Many foods have a combination of both types of fiber—for example, when you eat an apple, you're getting insoluble fiber from the skin and soluble fiber from the flesh. It's the best of both worlds, which is why I've been known to chomp down an apple while sitting in LA traffic or bustin' it in my trailer before hitting the stage to host a show!

SOURCES OF fiber

- Berries
- Apples and pears
- Nuts and dried fruit
- Whole grains
- Beans

VITAMINS AND MINERALS

Vitamins and minerals come from a variety of foods. The ingredients in Dana's meal plans are the best of the best when it comes to their vitamin and mineral content. To help make sense of some of the main nutrient powerhouses, here are my top five vitamins and minerals and a little bit about why each is so important.

Vitamins

>>**Vitamin A** is vital for healthy skin, eyes, and bone development. Food sources of vitamin A are milk, cheese, fruit and veggies like carrots, sweet potatoes, and leafy greens (such as spinach, kale, and Swiss chard).

>>**Vitamin C**, found in citrus fruits, potatoes, broccoli, strawberries, and bell peppers, helps maintain skin and connective tissue. It also helps the body absorb iron and fight inflammation.

>>You can't have strong bones or teeth without **vitamin D** from dairy products and fish. Your body also makes some of its own vitamin D from exposure to sunlight.

SOURCES OF
dairy

- Nonfat milk
- Low fat cheese
- Nonfat yogurt
- Cottage cheese
- Low fat buttermilk

>>**Vitamin E** helps protect cells from damage that can cause heart disease and certain types of cancer. Get vitamin E from whole grains, eggs, leafy green vegetables, and vegetable oils.

>>**B vitamins** like thiamin, riboflavin, and niacin are all involved in different stages of energy production, while vitamin B6 aids in protein metabolism. Vitamins B12 and folate play a role in DNA formation and production of healthy red blood cells. Lean meats and fish are loaded with various B vitamins, and some can also be found in whole grains, dairy, fruits, and vegetables.

Minerals

>>**Calcium** and **vitamin D** work together to form strong, healthy bones. Calcium is also important for proper muscle function. Dairy, beans, leafy greens, and calcium-fortified foods are all good ways to get your calcium.

>>Blood relies on **iron** to help carry oxygen throughout the body—pretty important, right? Meats, fish, legumes, whole grains, nuts, spinach, broccoli, and dried fruit are all good ways to get your iron.

>>**Potassium** is involved in muscle contraction and energy transport throughout the body to help keep you lean and your metabolism running high. Food sources include bananas, citrus fruits, milk, vegetables, meat, and fish.

>> You can't build strong and lean muscles or healthy bones without **magnesium**. Milk, yogurt, beans, nuts, whole grains, fruits, and vegetables are all good sources.

>>**Zinc** is critical for a properly functioning metabolism as well as a strong immune system. Get zinc from meats, fish, dairy, nuts, whole grains, and vegetables.

ANTIOXIDANTS

Antioxidants have a very important job: They protect cells from all kinds of wear and tear damage caused by harmful substances called free radicals. The best sources of antioxidants are brightly colored fruits and vegetables, whole grains, nuts, seeds, and legumes. Vitamins A, C, and E have antioxidant power, and there are hundreds of others that work in different parts of the body. Check out the meal plans and recipes (pages 37–216) where Dana and I have highlighted some of the antioxidants and how they work.

SOURCES OF
antioxidants

- Berries
- Leafy greens (kale, spinach, Swiss chard, and mixed greens)
- Beans
- Nuts and seeds
- Tomatoes

WATER

What you drink is just as important as what you eat. And just like not eating enough calories can zap your energy, dehydration can lead to fatigue too. All the metabolic functions in the body rely on water to function, including regulation of body temperature, digestion, and protection of vital organs.

Believe it or not, all fluids and foods contribute to your body's hydration, not just water. The best way to make sure you're adequately hydrated is to monitor the color of your urine—if it's pale in color or clear, you're getting enough. If it's dark yellow, you're not. But don't wait until you are thirsty to drink something—regular fluid intake should be part of your healthy lifestyle. I know that staying hydrated can be difficult, especially if you're exercising frequently, so here are some simple tips to make sure you're meeting your needs.

>>Carry something to drink with you at all times—even a few extra sips will make a difference.

- >>Eat plenty of fresh fruits and vegetables. This will benefit overall health and provide a significant amount of fluid.
- >>Monitor your sweat rate. The more sweat lost during an activity, the more fluid that needs to be replaced afterward.
- >>All fluids help to keep you hydrated, but water is best because it's absorbed quickly and is calorie free.

learn the importance of variety

Variety is an important component in the act of balancing your daily nutrients. If you eat the same foods every day, even if you're making healthy choices, you're limiting yourself to only those nutrients in those foods and missing out on other important nutrients that your body needs to be efficient. However, eating different foods and thus ensuring that all three macronutrients (carbs, protein, and fat) are represented at every major meal means you are creating a long-lasting, sustainable environment for your body to burn fat and perform at its best. In the seven-week meal plan section of this book, you will see that Dana has designed the meals to amount to the optimal balance of about one-half carbs, one-fourth protein, and one-fourth fat per day. In these seven weeks, you will condition your body and mind to naturally achieve this balance every day through a variety of healthy and tasty foods.

Remember, eating well shouldn't be about deprivation; rather, it should be about finding balance and variety and giving your body the exact amount of nutrients to perform at its best.

STEP 2.

practice proper portion control

THE BEST WAY to regulate your metabolism and maintain a fat-burning body is to take in a consistent amount of calories each day. The best way to keep calories under control is to keep portions under control. When you first dig into the meal plans and recipes you may need to keep the measuring cups and spoons handy for a little while, but eventually you'll be able to estimate portions automatically. Measuring out portions in the beginning can really help give you a sense of how much food you should be eating. So, going forward, whether you're cooking a favorite family recipe or ordering at a restaurant, you'll know how much food is right for you.

In the meal plans, you're going to see a lot of specific measurements and portion sizes of foods that you'll need to adhere to—two cups of mixed greens, four ounces of salmon, two tablespoons of cashews, etc. And all these numbers may seem overwhelming at first, especially if you're not used to measuring your food, but trust me, with a little due diligence right off the bat, picking the right portion sizes will become second nature before you know it. It will even get to the point where you won't need to measure anything; you'll be able to eyeball it and know exactly how much to eat at every meal.

Eating the proper portion sizes of foods at each and every meal is one of the most important aspects to any weight loss plan, so becoming familiar with how big the pile of rice or pasta should be, or how much space your lean steak should take up on your plate, is crucial. If your portion sizes are too big, you'll consume excess calories, which will not only keep you from losing weight, but will make you gain unwanted pounds too.

The first step to moderating your portion sizes is to look at the food label that's on the package of virtually every food you buy at the grocery. Now, these labels aren't exactly a "one size fits all" recommendation, but they'll at least offer a good starting point. "If you know how many calories are in a half cup of something," says Dana, "then you can determine if you need more or less of that food." This is especially helpful for the times when you're not following the meal plans directly; in this case, you'll know how many calories to eat at each meal (even when you're not following the meal plans in this book to a T, you should still be aiming for the same calorie totals and macronutrient ratios) and can use the food labels to help you hit your marks.

what to look for in food labels

- Check the serving size so you know what a proper portion should be
- When it comes to fat, choose foods that are low in saturated fat and free of trans fats; look for healthy mono and polyunsaturated fats
- Even if a food has fewer than 0.5 grams of fat per serving, the label can read 0 grams—check ingredient list for these "hidden" fats
- Choose high fiber grains, breads, and cereals—look for foods with three grams or more of fiber per serving
- Choose foods without processed sweeteners like high fructose corn syrup
- Choose foods without trans fats—they'll be listed as "partially hydrogenated" oils on the ingredient list
- Make sure grains are "whole" (whole wheat, whole grain oats, etc.)

- Added sugars go by many names: corn syrup, molasses, evaporated cane juice, brown sugar, invert sugar, just to name a few; these are the ones to avoid
- Avoid high-sodium processed foods like frozen dinners and packaged snacks
- If you don't recognize an ingredient, look it up!

When you're at home preparing your meals, such tools of the trade as measuring cups and spoons and even a food scale are all very wise investments. The measuring cups will help you determine the right amounts of salad, pasta, and rice (among other foods); measuring spoons will be especially helpful with salad dressings and cooking oils; and the food scale will come in handy with meats, like when you're trying to figure out how big a four-ounce tenderloin is supposed to be.

"Practice makes perfect," says Dana. "Once you measure something a few times, you begin to learn to recognize what a proper portion looks like. Being able to properly measure food also helps you cook, follow recipes, and order at restaurants—all skills necessary for a healthy lifestyle."

But when you're not at home—assuming you don't leave the house with your measuring cups—you may just need to eyeball it to determine proper portion sizes, especially if you're still new to the meal plans. For this, Dana has provided a list of visual cues to help you pick out the right size of food when your cooking tools aren't exactly handy. Each visual cue represents an item that can be found in the kitchen. Use this guide as your own personal "cheat sheet" to pick the right portion sizes:

MEATS, FISH, POULTRY

3 ounces = spatula head

SALAD DRESSING, PEANUT BUTTER

2 Tbsp = a lime

VEGETABLES

1 cup = a regular-sized apple

FRUIT

1 medium piece = a regular-sized apple 

1 small piece = a lime

½ cup berries = a pear

CHEESE

1 ounce = an ice cube

NUTS

¼ cup = a lime 

GRAINS

1 cup of popcorn or cereal = a regular-sized apple 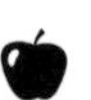

½ cup cooked rice = a lime

STEP 3.

eat frequently throughout the day

MONITORING THE FREQUENCY of how much you eat and what you eat throughout the day can seem like a daunting task. Who has the time to keep track of that kind of dietary schedule when your plate is already full—namely with your kids, spouse, and career? On the other hand, you know that the only way to balance your life efficiently is to be focused and have the energy to get through the day. When and how often you eat is just as important as *what* you eat. Since food gives you energy, you'll want to keep those energy levels high all day by eating small, frequent meals. Fatigue happens when the body doesn't have calories and fluid readily available, and most people don't eat enough during the day. Many factors may influence this, but the bottom line is that you must take action to prevent this from happening or your metabolism will pay the price. Many people end up trying to fit all the calories they need into a small portion of the day (usually in the evening). This is not efficient for the body's metabolism and will result in overeating and decreased performance when it comes to burning fat. So how can you keep this from happening? An even distribution of nutrients from meals and snacks all day long. This third step, eating frequently throughout the day, conditions your body to burn fat constantly by challenging your metabolism and keeping it revved up. And as with many things, planning and timing must be factored in when taking in your meals.

how food and exercise contribute to a more efficient metabolism

There's no big secret to weight loss. All it really comes down to is calories in and calories out. When you eat more calories than you burn, you gain weight; when you burn more calories than you eat, you lose it. The tricky part is learning how to do this effectively for the long haul, and it doesn't mean that you should eat nothing and exercise a lot to lose weight successfully. Eating the proper amount of calories from the correct ratio of macronutrients, vitamins, and minerals, along with a smart exercise regimen, is how you lose weight and keep it off for good.

When people go on crash diets and eat practically nothing, they may lose some weight, but since the body can't function on too little calories for very long, the weight always comes back. Taking drastic measures to drop weight only to gain it back is not only emotionally frustrating but also damaging to your metabolism. When you try to get by on too few calories, your metabolism slows down to compensate for the lack of energy. This means you're using calories less efficiently and, worst of all, you're left tired and hungry. When you eat the proper amount of calories and the right distribution of macronutrients, you allow for all proper chemical reactions to take place in the body, leading to energy production, muscle function, and a supercharged metabolism. Throw some exercise into the picture to boost metabolism even further and you've got everything you need to reach your goals. The bottom line is eating high quality nutrients from delicious foods along with exercise to keep your metabolism working efficiently.

the seven windows of opportunity

In my line of work, I'm always busy. I'm either constantly on-set or I'm traveling. Because of this, I'm faced with many decisions when it comes to eating, especially considering that many of my food options are at restaurants and aren't always very healthy. But through the years, I've learned how to make sure that I'm constantly eating and making good decisions even when I could've very easily gone the other direction. What has kept me on track and disciplined is finding seven quick windows throughout the day to nourish my body. In each of these moments, I also make sure to make smart decisions on what and how much I eat by balancing my daily intake of carbs, protein, and fat and staying within the proper portions. Taking advantage of these seven crucial windows of opportunity on a consistent basis has been the lifestyle I've led for many years now, and as a result, my metabolism is at an optimal state of efficiency.

Here are the seven windows of the day that you should use to practice long-lasting healthy habits when it comes to food and eating:

BREAKFAST

With breakfast being the first meal of the day and your body more or less coming off starvation mode from sleeping, it's really important to get your metabolism revved back up to start burning maximum calories and fat. That's the first reason why eating at this time is critical, so it's worth repeating: Don't skip breakfast.

That said, you really want to make sure that all macronutrients (carbs, protein, and fat) are represented first thing in the morning, because the second purpose of breakfast is to fuel for the first few hours of the day, until it's time to eat again. Practicing Step 1 (balancing your carbs, protein, and fat intake) at breakfast will do just that for one simple reason: digestion. Macronutrients are digested in a certain order: carbs are usually burned first, followed by protein and fat. If you have only, say, carbs at breakfast, after those have

FOODS TO BOOST metabolism

- Water
- Yogurt
- Almonds
- Berries
- Apples
- Leafy greens
- Lean meats
- Beans
- Oatmeal
- Soy

digested, there will be nothing left and you'll get hungry again prematurely. But if you have protein and fat to eat along with the carbs, those will continue to digest until right about the time you eat your first snack of the day (more on that meal shortly). The goal with breakfast, and any other meal for that matter, is to satisfy your immediate hunger as well as keep you satisfied and satiated until your next meal.

And when it comes to carbs, you want to make sure you're starting your day with whole grain choices like oatmeal, whole grain cereal, or whole grain toast. These will be your carb staples in the morning, though fruits and vegetables are also good, whether it means making a fresh fruit smoothie or mixing some vegetables in with your scrambled eggs. These are all great choices for providing your body the vitamins and minerals it needs, as well as satisfying your hunger to help keep you from overeating.

And beware (not just at breakfast, but most other times of the day as well) of "sugary" carbohydrates like Pop-Tarts, sugary cereals, and non–whole grain cereal bars. These foods are very popular these days, but they aren't wise choices. These types of carbs are essentially empty calories, meaning you're not really getting much out of them other than fast-burning calories. They're going to be digested really quickly and you're going to be left hungry very shortly after that. It's amazing how fast sugary snacks can get through your system—five minutes later you're already hungry! Besides that, these foods usually don't contain the fiber and vitamins that whole grain foods provide.

SUGARY FOODS to avoid

- Candy
- Cookies and cakes
- Store-bought muffins and pastries
- Soda
- Premade coffee drinks
- Drink mixes like iced tea and lemonade
- Regular peanut butter
- Many breakfast cereals
- Some bottled salad dressings

Speaking of fiber, I really think this is one of the secrets to weight control. Fiber is great for the obvious reasons but also because it makes you feel full, which means you'll be less likely to want to keep eating. It's recommended that we get between twenty and thirty grams of fiber a day, with good sources of fiber being whole grains, oatmeal, beans, and many fruits. Twenty to thirty grams may not seem like much, but it is, making it very important to start your day off with a good dose of fiber. The earlier you can start getting your fiber in, the better chance you'll have of meeting your needs for the day. Fiber also helps lower cholesterol, so besides helping control hunger, it's also great for your overall health.

Carbs are certainly important early in the day, but don't forget about protein and fat. As I stated earlier, a balance of nutrients is key first thing in the morning, so you'll need to choose foods other than just whole grains and fruit. One of my favorite sources of both protein and fat is eggs. But before you go making an egg white omelet, remember that there's just about as much protein in the yolks as in the whites. The yolks are also where you're going to get some of your much-needed dietary fat, not to mention other vitamins. Again, just like fiber, fat and protein are great for controlling hunger because of how slowly they digest. Protein is also necessary for maintaining muscle, which will keep your metabolism running higher, allowing you to burn more calories, even at rest.

A breakfast of eggs and oatmeal or whole grain toast is a great way to start your day. Two or three hours after, it'll be time to eat again.

MIDMORNING SNACK

I view snacks as my "bridges" between my main three meals of the day (breakfast, lunch, and dinner). But don't get me wrong, I consider snacks just as important as any other meal—no matter how small they are. When the goal is to eat small frequent meals throughout the day as a means of keeping your metabolism high and losing as much unwanted weight as possible, employing multiple snacks every day is the only way to achieve that. The midmorning snack is basically meant to carry you through those early hours of the day and keep your energy levels high between breakfast and lunch.

Like any other meal, the foods I choose when snacking are ones that won't be digested too quickly and will provide the body an abundance of nutrients, which means sugary snacks are pretty much always avoided. And even though you're eating less at these snacks—a general rule of thumb for the meal plans in this book is that all snacks are somewhere between seventy-five and one hundred and fifty calories—you still want them to be well-rounded with a variety of nutrients. Even if it's just a piece of fruit, you can still choose one that's higher in fiber (like an apple, pear, orange, or berries) to help slow down digestion and keep you satisfied for longer, at least until lunchtime.

And within that seventy-five to one hundred and fifty calorie range, you have some flexibility, which will be based off what you ate for breakfast. For example, let's say you had a fruit smoothie first thing in the morning but it was relatively low in calories. At your snack two to three hours later, feel free to have a more substantial amount of food at the upper end of the calorie range, around one hundred and fifty calories. On the other hand, if you have an omelet and a piece of toast for breakfast and it was relatively high in calories, a piece of fruit will be enough of a snack to tide you over for another couple of hours. Again, balance is the key, even at one of your smallest meals.

HEALTHY
snack foods

- Fresh fruit
- Carrot sticks and hummus
- Celery and peanut butter
- Part-skim mozzarella string cheese
- Nonfat yogurt
- Nuts
- Dried fruit
- Whole wheat pretzels
- Brown rice cakes
- Cottage cheese

Another good snack could be a granola bar. In it, you might have some dried fruit and whole grains, which will provide your carbohydrates, some nuts for healthy fats, and even a little bit of protein. So right there, in a simple granola bar, is a great balance of nutrients to keep you energized and your hunger level under control. Yogurt is also a great snack, as it contains carbs as well as protein from dairy. Even just a handful of almonds is a great source of fiber and dietary fat. The cool thing is, snacks don't necessarily have to be a combination of foods in order to provide a variety of nutrients. Sometimes one food will do it on its own.

LUNCH

By the middle of the day, assuming you've had your breakfast and snack, your metabolism should be running high and you'll want to continue that by putting some more fuel in the tank, so to speak. A lot of people will get busy at work and will skip lunch, and that's where they'll get into trouble. When you do this, your energy levels will start to take a nosedive—not to mention being hungry will negatively affect your concentration at work. The snack you had a couple of hours earlier was fairly small, so with lunch you'll want something more substantial. Where macronutrients are concerned, your lunch should more or less emulate breakfast with a good combination of healthy carbs, protein, and healthy fat, even though your food choices will likely be different—most people don't want to eat eggs and oatmeal for lunch.

At this point of the day, think back to the macronutrient ratio: about one-half of daily calories from carbohydrates, about one-fourth from fat, and about one-fourth from protein. Again, keep in mind that not every meal will contain this ratio; rather, this encompasses the entire day. (Snacks, in particular, will sometimes be more heavily weighted in one nutrient or another.) Because of this, Dana and I have balanced out carbohydrate intake between lunch and dinner in the meal plans with the intent of hitting that daily target of carbs and not exceeding it. To put it simply, the higher lunch is in carbs, the lower your dinner will be in carbs. At the same time, if carbs are low at lunch, they'll be a little higher at dinner.

For example, if you have a sandwich for lunch that includes whole grain bread, your dinner should probably be absent of rice, pasta, potatoes, or bread because you got enough of these types of foods at lunch. But if your lunch was lower in carbs—say, you had a salad—then dinner will be higher in carbs. And it's very important to note that when I talk about higher versus lower carb intake at these two meals, I'm mainly referring to starchy carbohydrates (potatoes, pasta, rice, etc.), not vegetables. Your lunch or dinner might not contain any of these starches, but vegetables are definitely fair game.

This balance of carbs between lunch and dinner is exactly what I do almost every day. If my lunch consisted of chicken with broccoli, then I'll enjoy some pasta or rice for dinner. This is the flexibility I've been harping on throughout this book. You have the freedom to go a little higher in carbs at either lunch or dinner by simply keeping your carb intake strict at the other.

Dana and I even believe that alternating meals, lunch or dinner, higher in carbs on different days will increase the metabolism for more calorie burning. So instead of always having lunch as your higher carbs meal and dinner low, or vice versa, you should switch it up day to day. "By alternating in this fashion," says Dana, "I think it works more efficiently from a metabolic standpoint. It's a good way to balance things."

Lunch is also a common time for people to overeat, mainly because they choose to eat out at a restaurant, where portion sizes usually aren't friendly to the health-minded person. Not surprisingly, when you overeat you're likely to gain weight. How this works in the body is actually a very simple concept: At a given meal, your body uses what it needs from the food you eat for energy and other functions. Anything on top of that (the "surplus" calories and nutrients) often ends up being stored in the body as fat. When you overeat, your body doesn't know what to do with all those extra nutrients, so they get stored.

Which leads me to the types of foods you want to be eating at lunchtime, specifically protein. One reason protein is favored by those looking to lose weight is that it's not easily stored in the body. Most times, a slight surplus of protein simply leaves the body via excretion. Pretty great, huh? However, just like any nutrient, protein needs to be moderated. Even though it's not easily stored, protein *does* contain calories, and a vast surplus of them can in fact be stored as body fat.

When picking your protein source at lunch, cold cuts in sandwiches are a very common choice, though not always the best choice. If you must have cold cuts, look for low sodium deli turkey and chicken breast instead of roast beef and ham, which tend to be higher in fat. The low sodium isn't just about controlling blood pressure, since people not at risk for high blood pressure don't need to be as concerned with sodium intake as those at risk. Sodium intake in this case is more about water retention; high sodium foods (most deli meats, for example) will cause you to retain water, which you don't want. The best sources of protein at lunchtime are grilled chicken breast, beans, and even tofu, which is a great plant-based protein source that you'll see pop up occasionally as an option in the meal plan.

When it comes to carbs at lunch, I'm probably starting to sound like a broken record when I say always reach for whole grains, fruits, and vegetables, regardless of the time of day. Low fat dairy and beans also include good carbohydrates, in addition to protein, so they're great foods for lunch as well.

If you can stay focused at lunchtime and take advantage of this oh so important window of opportunity, you'll be fueled through much of the afternoon and your body will be burning fat the entire time.

LATE-AFTERNOON SNACK

The time between lunch and dinner can be a long one, which is why two midday snacks are provided in the meal plan. The purpose of these snacks is simply to keep your energy levels high as you finish out the workday or a fast-paced afternoon with the kids, but also to keep your metabolism running and to stave off hunger.

Of all the times during the day when people go long periods without eating, I think this one is the most common, and the most troublesome too. The worst thing you can do is eat lunch at noon and then eat nothing until seven o'clock when it's time for dinner. Early evening (right after work) is also the time when many people fit their exercise in, which further compounds the problem of not eating enough, since you'll be hungrier and will need that much more energy. When you don't eat for that long a period of time, you're setting yourself up for disaster to overeat that evening and into the night.

These snacks will each be small; you can even think of them as one regular-sized snack split into two separate snacks. This way, you're spreading out your meals even that much more to ensure that you never go long periods of time without eating, as a means of avoiding the tendency to eat *anything in sight* near the end of your workday—because often times, "anything in sight" means eating something unhealthy from a vending machine at the office. By eating these snacks, you're also avoiding that dreaded "afternoon crash," when low energy levels make you want to take a nap at your desk.

The types of foods you'll be eating here will be very similar to those of your midmorning snack—foods that will provide energy through good carbs and fend off hunger with good amounts of fiber and even healthy fat. For example, a serving of string cheese and an orange is a typical snack. With the two midday meals, you'll eat, say, the string cheese, then have the orange an hour or two later. These snacks aren't going to be that far apart, so they're kind of working together even though you're not eating them at the same time. You're creating that combination of foods and nutrients even though there may be an hour or two in between eating them. Doing this will also help keep you occupied and not thinking about eating something unhealthy in your downtime.

One thing I love about these midday snacks is that they fit a busy lifestyle perfectly. If you have a meeting at two thirty and have little time to eat, all it takes is eating an apple or a handful of almonds on the way there. Then, when it's over, you can eat another snack, like a serving of yogurt. Some might see such small meals as limiting, but I see them as being very conducive to a busy, on-the-go work schedule. It also works great for mothers who stay at home and don't have time to cook a lot of meals. When you have a few minutes of spare time (like when the kids are napping), grab a piece of fruit or some nuts. These meals are both flexible and interchangeable. From the above example, if you'd prefer to eat the string cheese for the first of two snacks, and then the orange, that's fine. But if you'd rather eat the orange first, that'll work too.

The second of these two snacks will also work well for those who tend to snack as they fix dinner. I talk to a lot of people who say they can't stop picking at food as they cook, to the point where they've eaten a full meal's worth of calories before they even sit down to dinner. But if you can have a small snack right when you get home from work (say, at around five or six o'clock), that should curb your hunger until dinner is served just an hour or two later.

FOODS TO
curb cravings

- Cottage cheese
- Beans
- Nonfat yogurt
- Dried fruit
- Fresh fruit
- Peanut butter
- Trail mix
- Whole grain cereal
- Air-popped popcorn
- Brown rice cakes

Again, sugary carbs that won't satisfy your hunger aren't a wise choice at these two meals. In that large window of opportunity between lunch and dinner, you'll need to choose foods that fill you up and keep you going. In this four-, five- or seven-hour period, you'll often find that there are two crucial moments when you'll need to make the right decision. Do this and you'll set yourself up for success at dinner and later in the evening.

DINNER

Dinner is a time when many people overeat. But I hope that some of that will be minimized by the simple fact that you've followed through on the previous five meals and snacks and aren't as hungry as normal come dinnertime. Because even though people tend to overeat by the end of the day, many of us don't eat nearly enough early in the day, which leads to overeating at night. Think about it: How many times have you told someone, "All I've had to eat today was a bowl of cereal and a bagel," or whatever the foods happened to be. By doing this, you've created two problems. First, you're so hungry at night that you overeat, and second, your lack of eating early in the day didn't allow your metabolism to run high. By skipping multiple meals in the morning and afternoon, you've missed opportunities to burn calories and fat during the day.

If you've followed Step 1 throughout the day, you'll see that simply balancing your meals will help manage your diet overall. There's a common misconception that carbs eaten at night will be stored as fat more so than carbs eaten in the afternoon. True, carbs you eat for dinner can very easily be stored as fat, but it's not simply because of what your watch says. As long as by the end of the day you've met your calorie and macronutrient needs (neither exceeding nor falling short of them) and you've spaced your food intake out evenly during the day, you'll be fine.

Where people run into trouble is when they eat a high carb lunch and then eat a bunch of starchy carbs at dinner—for example, bread on a sandwich at noon and a large serving of pasta six hours later. There's a good chance that with that sandwich and subsequent snacks you've practically met your carbohydrate needs, at least where starches are concerned. So if you proceed to eat more carbs at dinner, then yes, the more of them you eat the worse off you'll be from a metabolic and weight loss standpoint. On the flip side, if you're short on carbs and calories at six or seven o'clock, you're doing the right thing by having some healthy carbs with dinner. As you will see, this is the whole reason why Dana balances out the carbs you eat between lunch and dinner in the meal plan.

If you have a salad with grilled chicken and vegetables (something low in starchy carbs) for lunch, at dinner you can get away with a reasonable portion of rice, whole grain pasta or bread, or even one of Dana's pizza recipes she worked into the meal plan. If you see a dinner in the meal plan that doesn't contain a lot of carbs—only vegetables, with the focus more on protein and healthy fat—it's not just because the sun has gone down; it's because your carbs were on the high end early in the day.

This balancing act between lunch and dinner, especially where carbs are concerned, is a critical element to making this meal plan, and any other meal plan for that matter, work for you. Lunch will orchestrate what you have for dinner more than breakfast will. Because breakfast is always about jump-starting your metabolism after not having eaten anything throughout the night, you can tend to go a little heavier on the carbs, since your body needs the energy.

Choosing what to eat for dinner can either be dependent on what you've eaten up to that point, and then filling in the holes so to speak, or you can plan your dinner and work backward from there. In other words, dinner shouldn't always be what you're left with for the day. It will take a little more planning on the front end, but you'll find that such planning will become second nature.

Where most people get into trouble in terms of carbs is with portion sizes. You'll notice in Dana's meal plans that one cup of pasta or a half cup of cooked rice is specified. Many of you are probably used to larger serving sizes of starchy carbs, but as you'll learn through the meal plans, those large portions are not only unnecessary but counterproductive.

Obviously, protein will be a major part of dinner, and the meal plan does a great job of introducing all kinds of different sources, from pork chops and turkey burgers and vegetarian chili to salmon. In most of these types of foods, you're also getting a good amount of healthy fat, which, as you know, is a key nutrient to keep balanced throughout the day because of how slowly it digests. You don't want your dinner to digest too quickly (otherwise you'll be hungry an hour later), but that's what will happen if you neglect including healthy fat in that meal.

And even though your workday is probably over by the time you eat dinner, it's still important to end the day with a good, well-rounded meal. Everything you do requires calories for energy. Even when you're sleeping, you're always using energy. Plus remember, overnight is the longest you'll go without eating so it's important to provide your body with lasting health for the overnight fast. If you don't eat enough for dinner, you're setting yourself up for an energy deficit later on. By skimping on dinner, you're creating a longer period of not eating, which can lead to overeating later on—maybe not that night, but the next day or the day after, for sure.

BEFORE-BEDTIME SNACK

This time of the day is different from the previous six because it's the one moment where you don't really need to eat, provided you've gotten the rest of your meals in to that point. You'll see in the meal plan that you do have the option to eat one more small snack. The rule of thumb here is simple: If you're hungry, eat the snack; if you're not hungry, don't eat it.

This is really the time of day when you should be asking yourself, "Am I really hungry or is it just a habit for me to eat late at night?" If the latter applies, you're better off skipping the meal. Either way, this sixty-calorie (or so) snack won't make or break your nutrient ratio or calorie needs, so feel free to enjoy this small indulgence, which will typically take on the form of a dessert-like food and provide a quick sweet fix. Some examples of this snack include half a frozen banana, some pineapple, or sugar-free gelatin.

When it comes down to it, the six small, well-balanced meals you've eaten up to this point will leave you at a place where further calories and macronutrient consumption is unnecessary. And eating a full meal at this point will likely push you over your calorie target and possibly lead to weight gain, so stick to only a low calorie snack. But remember, this isn't because of some golden rule that says anything eaten after, say, seven or eight o'clock at night will be stored as fat. The body doesn't really work that way. Weight gain is calorie sensitive, not time sensitive. It just so happens that typically by the end of the day you've already achieved sufficient calorie intake and any more could result in a surplus.

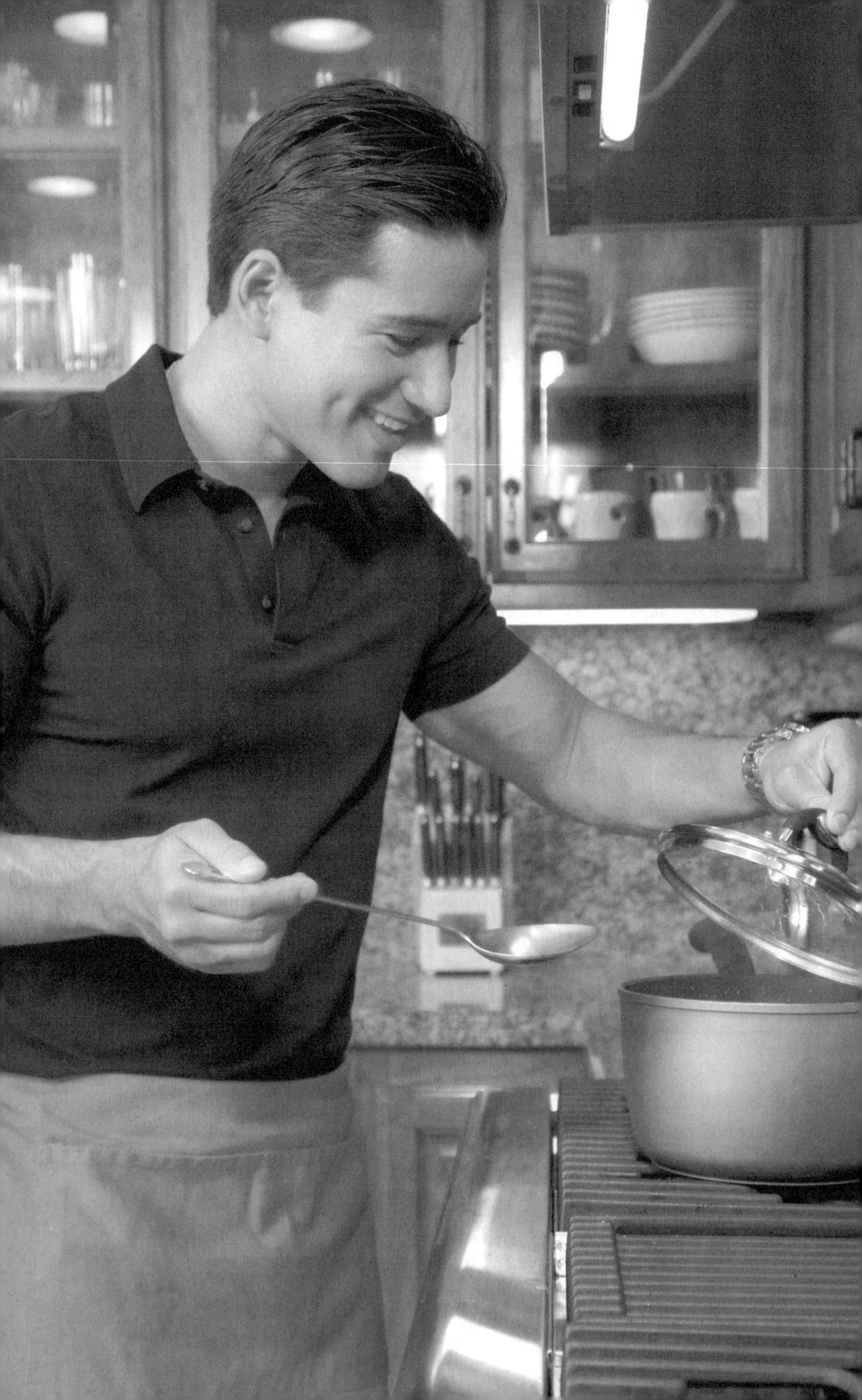

live extra lean every day

SECTION 2

NOW THAT YOU'VE learned how to condition your body to burn fat at the most optimum level, the focus can be on delicious food and implementing the three rules. Each day will contain the optimal health and fat-burning ratios of all macronutrients. Carbohydrate intake will comprise about one-half of your calories, dietary fat one-fourth of calories, and about one-fourth for protein. Remember, balance is the key to creating the proper conditions for your body to burn fat efficiently. Carbohydrates, fat, and protein all need to be represented adequately every day to allow for sustained energy for both work and exercise, as well as to keep hunger under control.

Each meal contains just the right amount of food to keep you sustained and to help curb cravings. These portions also ensure that your caloric count is in check, so you're guaranteed to shed pounds simply by cutting down calories at each meal.

This meal plan includes six to seven portioned meals per day so that you are conditioned to eat frequently throughout the day. Eating the right foods in the right amounts will lead to an increased metabolism and fat-burning body.

Finally, the foods selected for this plan are accessible, nutritious, and absolutely delicious. I don't believe in eating foods that I will not enjoy, so all meals reflect taste just as much as health. You need to enjoy good food to have long-lasting health and permanent weight loss, and this meal plan will show you how.

MEAL PLANS

the **extra** lean

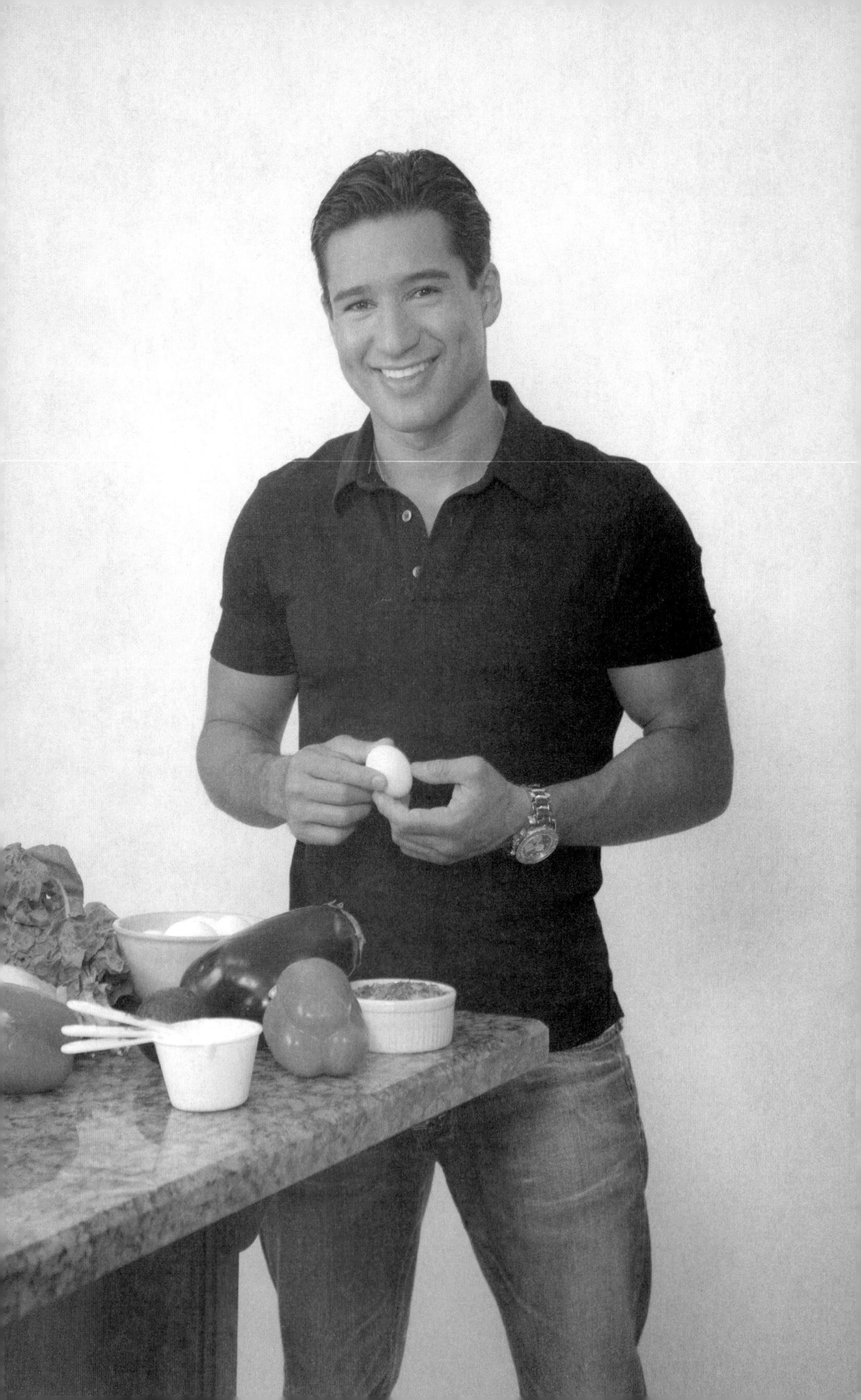

BREAKFAST

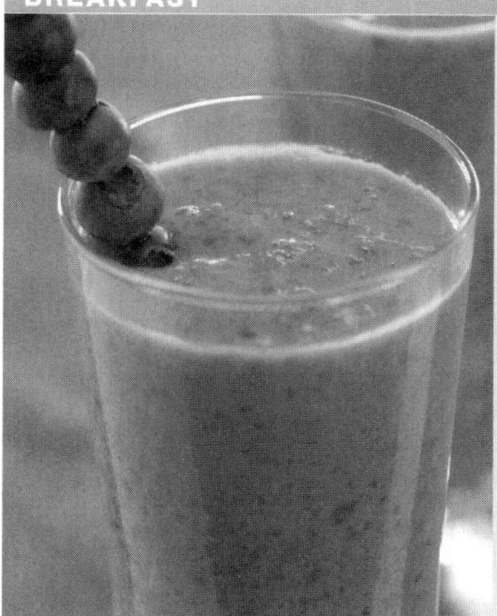

▸ Berry Blast Smoothie

SERVES: 1

1 cup frozen mixed berries
½ cup nonfat vanilla yogurt
½ cup orange juice
¼ cup water

Place ingredients into a blender and blend until smooth.

Calories: 188 kcal
Total Fat: 0.5 g
Saturated Fat: 0 g
Total Carbohydrate: 42 g
Protein: 6 g
Sodium: 80 mg
Fiber: 3 g

NUTRIENT INTAKE:

84% carbs
14% protein
2% fat

SNACK 1

▸ 10 almonds

Calories: 69 kcal
Total Fat: 6 g
Saturated Fat: 0.5 g
Total Carbohydrate: 2 g
Protein: 3 g
Sodium: 0 mg
Fiber: 1 g

NUTRIENT INTAKE:

13% carbs
14% protein
73% fat

LUNCH

▸ Spinach Salad with Grapes and Grilled Chicken

2 cups baby spinach
½ cup sliced cucumber
¼ cup grapes, halved
3 oz grilled chicken breast, sliced
1 Tbsp white wine vinegar
2 tsp extra-virgin olive oil

Baby spinach—swap out lettuce for leafy greens like spinach for salads and sandwiches for extra vitamins and minerals

Calories: 282 kcal
Total Fat: 12 g
Saturated Fat: 2 g
Total Carbohydrate: 13 g
Protein: 30 g
Sodium: 157 mg
Fiber: 3 g

NUTRIENT INTAKE:
19% carbs
42% protein
39% fat

SNACK 2

- 1 medium banana

Calories: 105 kcal
Total Fat: 0 g
Saturated Fat: 0 g
Total Carbohydrate: 27 g
Protein: 1 g
Sodium: 1 mg
Fiber: 3 g

NUTRIENT INTAKE:
57% carbs
16% protein
27% fat

SNACK 3

- 6 whole wheat crackers
- 1 part-skim mozzarella string cheese

Calories: 140 kcal
Total Fat: 7.5 g
Saturated Fat: 3.5 g
Total Carbohydrate: 11 g
Protein: 9 g
Sodium: 360 mg
Fiber: 2 g

NUTRIENT INTAKE:
30% carbs
24% protein
46% fat

DINNER

- 4 oz salmon roasted with 1 tsp olive oil, salt and pepper
- 1 medium baked sweet potato
- 1 cup steamed broccoli

Calories: 406 kcal
Total Fat: 14 g
Saturated Fat: 2.5 g
Total Carbohydrate: 35 g
Protein: 37 g
Sodium: 165 mg
Fiber: 9 g

NUTRIENT INTAKE:
34% carbs
36% protein
30% fat

Salmon—packed with heart-healthy omega-3 fatty acids

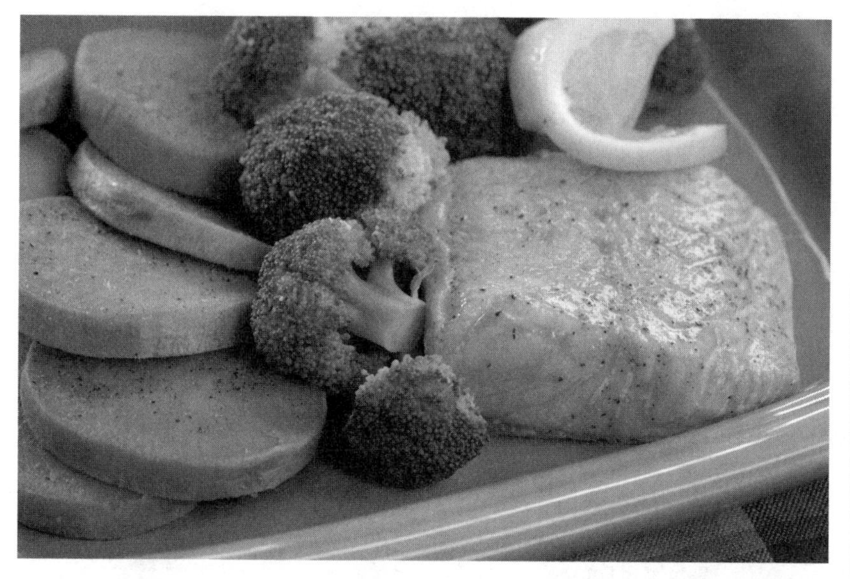

SNACK 4 (OPTIONAL)

▸ **1 cup air-popped popcorn**

Calories: 31 kcal
Total Fat: 0 g
Saturated Fat: 0 g
Total Carbohydrate: 6 g
Protein: 1 g
Sodium: 1 mg
Fiber: 1 g

NUTRIENT INTAKE:

77% carbs
13% protein
10% fat

NUTRITION FOR THE DAY

Calories: 1220 kcal
Total Fat: 41 g
Saturated Fat: 9 g
Total Carbohydrate: 136 g
Protein: 87 g
Sodium: 764 mg
Fiber: 23 g

NUTRIENT INTAKE:

45% carbs
23% protein
32% fat

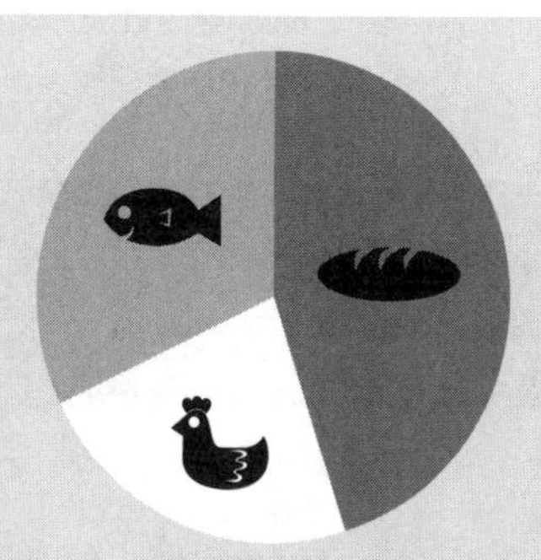

Remember to pay attention to the overall nutrient intake for the day. Adhere to Step 1 and aim for one-half carbs, one-quarter fats, one-quarter protein.

BREAKFAST

- **1 cup cooked oatmeal, topped with ½ tsp cinnamon, 1 tsp honey, and 1 Tbsp raisins**

Calories: 199 kcal
Total Fat: 2 g
Saturated Fat: 0 g
Total Carbohydrate: 39 g
Protein: 6 g
Sodium: 4 mg
Fiber: 5 g

NUTRIENT INTAKE:

77% carbs
13% protein
10% fat

SNACK 1

- **6 oz nonfat fruit or vanilla yogurt**

Calories: 130 kcal
Total Fat: 0 g
Saturated Fat: 0 g
Total Carbohydrate: 26 g
Protein: 6 g
Sodium: 105 mg
Fiber: 2 g

NUTRIENT INTAKE:

81% carbs
19% protein
0% fat

LUNCH

- **1 hard-boiled egg**
- **Chopped Greek Salad**

1 cup sliced cucumber
1 cup cherry tomatoes, halved
2 Tbsp crumbled low fat feta cheese
—save calories and saturated fat by choosing low fat cheeses
¼ cup sliced black olives
2 Tbsp light vinaigrette salad dressing

Low fat cheeses—save calories, saturated fat, and cholesterol by choosing low fat and part-skim cheese

Calories: 255 kcal
Total Fat: 16.5 g
Saturated Fat: 5 g
Total Carbohydrate: 14 g
Protein: 14 g
Sodium: 1077 mg
Fiber: 3 g

NUTRIENT INTAKE:

22% carbs
21% protein
57% fat

SNACK 2

- **1 medium orange**

Calories: 62 kcal
Total Fat: 0 g
Saturated Fat: 0 g
Total Carbohydrate: 15 g
Protein: 1 g
Sodium: 0 mg
Fiber: 3 g

NUTRIENT INTAKE:

90% carbs
8% protein
2% fat

SNACK 3

- **10 celery strips**
- **1 Tbsp natural peanut butter—no added sugars or oils**

Natural peanut butter—contains no added sugars or extra oils; look for a brand that contains only peanuts and salt

Calories: 111 kcal
Total Fat: 8 g
Saturated Fat: 1 g
Total Carbohydrate: 4 g
Protein: 4 g
Sodium: 92 mg
Fiber: 2 g

NUTRIENT INTAKE:

16% carbs
16% protein
68% fat

DINNER

Turkey and Black Bean Burrito

SERVES: 1

1 tsp canola oil
4 oz ground turkey breast
2 Tbsp diced red onion
¼ cup diced red bell pepper
¼ tsp chili powder
¼ tsp cumin
1 Tbsp barbecue sauce
Pinch kosher salt
1 tsp freshly squeezed lime juice
¼ cup canned black beans (rinsed and drained)
1 (8 inch) whole wheat flour tortilla
¼ cup mixed greens
2 Tbsp shredded low fat cheddar cheese
Hot sauce (optional)

1. Heat oil in a skillet over medium heat—add turkey meat and sauté until browned.
2. Add onion and pepper; season with chili powder, cumin, barbecue sauce, salt, and lime juice. Sauté for an additional 5 to 7 minutes. Add beans and heat through.
3. Place turkey mixture in tortilla, top with greens, cheese, and hot sauce, roll up and enjoy.

Calories: 426 kcal
Total Fat: 10 g
Saturated Fat: 1 g
Total Carbohydrate: 40 g
Protein: 40 g
Sodium: 836 mg
Fiber: 8 g

NUTRIENT INTAKE:

39% carbs

39% protein

22% fat

SNACK 4 (OPTIONAL)

- **1 plum or tangerine**

Calories: 30 kcal
Total Fat: 0 g
Saturated Fat: 0 g
Total Carbohydrate: 8 g
Protein: 0 g
Sodium: 0 mg
Fiber: 1 g

NUTRIENT INTAKE:

90% carbs

5% protein

5% fat

NUTRITION FOR THE DAY

Calories: 1212 kcal
Total Fat: 37 g
Saturated Fat: 7.5 g
Total Carbohydrate: 146 g
Protein: 74 g
Sodium: 2114 mg
Fiber: 24 g

NUTRIENT INTAKE:

59% carbs

17% protein

23% fat

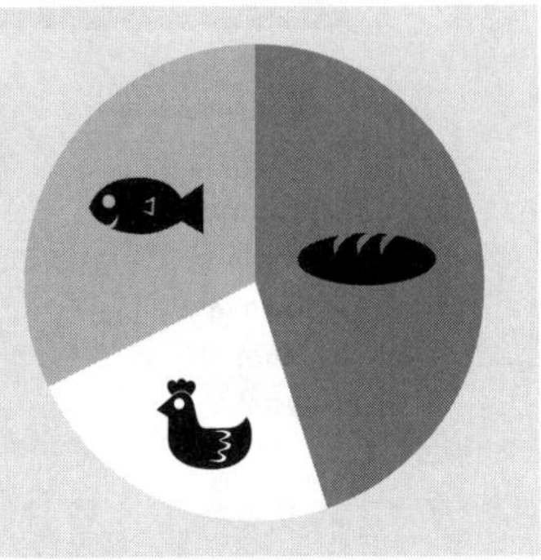

BREAKFAST

- **2 eggs, scrambled with ½ cup chopped tomato and ¼ cup diced low sodium turkey breast**
- **1 slice whole wheat toast**

Calories: 333 kcal
Total Fat: 12.5 g
Saturated Fat: 3.5 g
Total Carbohydrate: 24 g
Protein: 30 g
Sodium: 645 mg
Fiber: 4 g

NUTRIENT INTAKE:

29% carbs
37% protein
34% fat

SNACK 1

- **10 strawberries**

Calories: 58 kcal
Total Fat: 0.5 g
Saturated Fat: 0 g
Total Carbohydrate: 14 g
Protein: 1 g
Sodium: 2 mg
Fiber: 4 g

NUTRIENT INTAKE:

85% carbs
8% protein
7% fat

LUNCH

Brown Rice Salad

SERVES: 1

2 tsp extra-virgin olive oil
2 tsp freshly squeezed lemon juice
½ tsp Dijon mustard
½ tsp honey
Salt and pepper to taste
¾ cup cooked brown rice
½ cup chopped tomato
¼ cup chopped celery
¼ cup canned black beans (rinsed and drained)
1 Tbsp chopped fresh parsley

In a medium bowl, combine olive oil, lemon juice, mustard, and honey; season with salt and pepper and whisk well to combine. Add rice, tomato, celery, beans, and parsley, toss to combine.

Canned beans— always rinse and drain canned beans before using; this reduces up to 40% of the sodium.

Calories: 281 kcal
Total Fat: 10 g
Saturated Fat: 1.5 g
Total Carbohydrate: 41 g
Protein: 7 g
Sodium: 328 mg
Fiber: 8 g

NUTRIENT INTAKE:

57% carbs
11% protein
32% fat

SNACK 2

- 6 oz nonfat fruit or vanilla yogurt

Calories: 130 kcal
Total Fat: 0 g
Saturated Fat: 0 g
Total Carbohydrate: 26 g
Protein: 6 g
Sodium: 105 mg
Fiber: 2 g

NUTRIENT INTAKE:

81% carbs
19% protein
0% fat

SNACK 3

- 1 granola bar (Kashi)

Calories: 130 kcal
Total Fat: 5 g
Saturated Fat: 0.5 g
Total Carbohydrate: 20 g
Protein: 5 g
Sodium: 90 mg
Fiber: 4 g

NUTRIENT INTAKE:

68% carbs
16% protein
16% fat

Granola bars are an easy, portion controlled, on-the-go snack. Go for quality ingredients and choose a brand without a lot of added sugars.

DINNER

- 4 oz grilled chicken breast
- 1½ cups sliced zucchini roasted with 1 tsp olive oil

Calories: 254 kcal
Total Fat: 9 g
Saturated Fat: 2 g
Total Carbohydrate: 6 g
Protein: 37 g
Sodium: 101 mg
Fiber: 2 g

NUTRIENT INTAKE:

9% carbs
59% protein
32% fat

SNACK 4 (OPTIONAL)

▸ **10 baby carrots**

Calories: 35 kcal
Total Fat: 0 g
Saturated Fat: 0 g
Total Carbohydrate: 8 g
Protein: 1 g
Sodium: 78 mg
Fiber: 2 g

NUTRIENT INTAKE:

90% carbs
7% protein
3% fat

NUTRITION FOR THE DAY

Calories: 1221 kcal
Total Fat: 37.5 g
Saturated Fat: 7.5 g
Total Carbohydrate: 140 g
Protein: 88 g
Sodium: 1344 mg
Fiber: 25 g

NUTRIENT INTAKE:

60% carbs
22% protein
18% fat

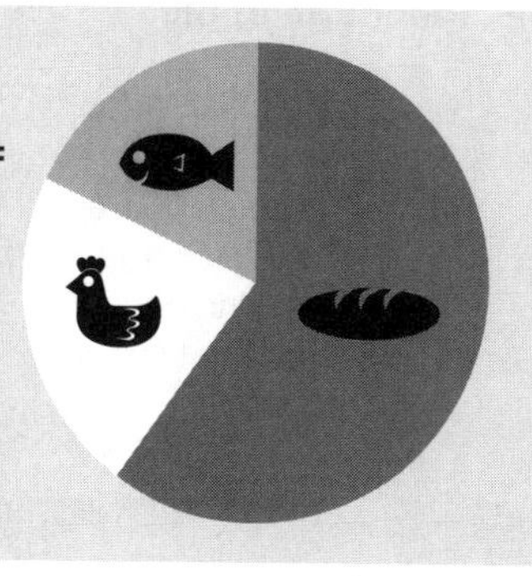

BREAKFAST

- 1 whole wheat English muffin, toasted with 1 Tbsp natural peanut butter
- 1 medium orange

Calories: 301 kcal
Total Fat: 9.5 g
Saturated Fat: 1.5 g
Total Carbohydrate: 45 g
Protein: 11 g
Sodium: 480 mg
Fiber: 9 g

NUTRIENT INTAKE:
58% carbs
14% protein
28% fat

SNACK 1

- 1 medium apple

Calories: 72 kcal
Total Fat: 0 g
Saturated Fat: 0 g
Total Carbohydrate: 19 g
Protein: 0 g
Sodium: 1 mg
Fiber: 3g

NUTRIENT INTAKE:
96% carbs
2% protein
2% fat

LUNCH

- 1 medium baked sweet potato topped with ½ cup steamed broccoli and 1 Tbsp nonfat Greek yogurt
- 1½ cups mixed greens with 1 Tbsp low fat vinaigrette

Calories: 174 kcal
Total Fat: 2.5 g
Saturated Fat: 0 g
Total Carbohydrate: 34 g
Protein: 6 g
Sodium: 336 mg
Fiber: 8 g

NUTRIENT INTAKE:
75% carbs
13% protein
12% fat

Greek yogurt—has a creamier texture and tangier flavor than regular yogurt—it's also higher in protein.

SNACK 2

- **10 baby carrots**
- **¼ cup hummus**

Calories: 128 kcal
Total Fat: 5.5 g
Saturated Fat: 1 g
Total Carbohydrate: 16 g
Protein: 5 g
Sodium: 290 mg
Fiber: 5 g

NUTRIENT INTAKE:

48% carbs
15% protein
37% fat

SNACK 3

- **10 unsalted almonds**
- **2 oz low sodium turkey breast**

Calories: 129 kcal
Total Fat: 6.5 g
Saturated Fat: 0.5 g
Total Carbohydrate: 2 g
Protein: 15 g
Sodium: 340 mg
Fiber: 1 g

NUTRIENT INTAKE:

7% carbs
46% protein
47% fat

DINNER

Beef Stir-Fry

SERVES: 1

Like it hot? Add a dash of chili sauce for some extra spice.

1 tsp canola oil
4 oz thinly sliced flank steak
1 clove garlic, minced
1 tsp grated fresh ginger root
1 cup chopped broccoli
1 cup diced red bell pepper
½ cup sliced red onion
1 Tbsp reduced sodium soy sauce
1 Tbsp teriyaki or hoisin sauce

1. Heat oil in a skillet or wok over medium-high heat, add beef and cook for 1 minute.
2. Add garlic, ginger, broccoli, pepper, and onion; cook, tossing continuously for 2 minutes.
3. Add soy sauce and teriyaki sauce and cook for an additional 1 to 2 minutes or until broccoli is crisp-tender.

Calories: 333 kcal
Total Fat: 11 g
Saturated Fat: 3 g
Total Carbohydrate: 30 g
Protein: 31 g
Sodium: 865 mg
Fiber: 4 g

NUTRIENT INTAKE:

35% carbs
36% protein
29% fat

SNACK 4 (OPTIONAL)

▸ **1 cup sugar-free, fat-free chocolate pudding**

Calories: 60 kcal
Total Fat: 1.5 g
Saturated Fat: 1 g
Total Carbohydrate: 14 g
Protein: 2 g
Sodium: 180 mg
Fiber: 1 g

NUTRIENT INTAKE:

72% carbs
11% protein
17% fat

NUTRITION FOR THE DAY

Calories: 1197 kcal
Total Fat: 37 g
Saturated Fat: 7 g
Total Carbohydrate: 161 g
Protein: 70 g
Sodium: 2393 mg
Fiber: 32 g

NUTRIENT INTAKE:

56% carbs
19% protein
25% fat

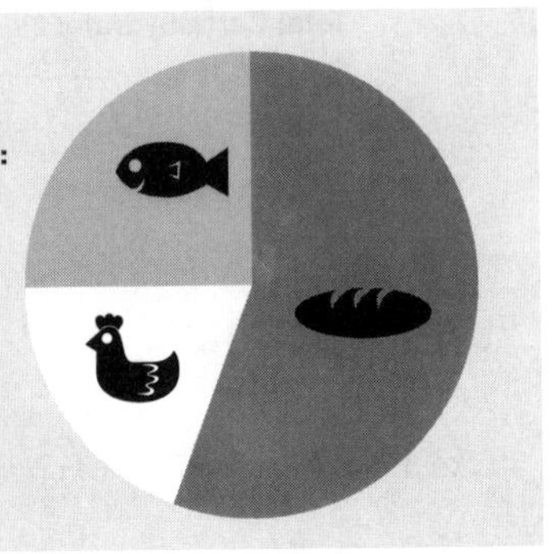

BREAKFAST

- 1 cup whole grain cereal (suggestions: Bran Flakes, Nature's Path Heirloom Flakes)
- ¾ cup skim milk
- ½ cup sliced strawberries

Calories: 219 kcal
Total Fat: 11 g
Saturated Fat: 1 g
Total Carbohydrate: 48 g
Protein: 11 g
Sodium: 371 mg
Fiber: 9 g

NUTRIENT INTAKE:

78% carbs

17% protein

5% fat

SNACK 1

- 1 part-skim mozzarella string cheese
- 2 oz low sodium turkey breast

Calories: 140 kcal
Total Fat: 7 g
Saturated Fat: 3.5 g
Total Carbohydrate: 1 g
Protein: 20 g
Sodium: 570 mg
Fiber: 0 g

NUTRIENT INTAKE:

3% carbs

54% protein

43% fat

LUNCH

- 1½ cups low sodium lentil soup (such as Amy's brand)
- 3 oz diced grilled chicken breast

Lentils—legumes like lentils, beans, and peas contain protein, healthy carbs, and fiber

Calories: 365 kcal
Total Fat: 9 g
Saturated Fat: 1.5 g
Total Carbohydrate: 35 g
Protein: 37 g
Sodium: 573 mg
Fiber: 9 g

NUTRIENT INTAKE:

38% carbs

40% protein

22% fat

SNACK 2

▸ **1 medium banana**

Calories: 105 kcal
Total Fat: 3.5 g
Saturated Fat: 0.5 g
Total Carbohydrate: 35 g
Protein: 4 g
Sodium: 122 mg
Fiber: 5 g

NUTRIENT INTAKE:

92% carbs
4% protein
4% fat

SNACK 3

▸ **1 cup sliced cucumber**
▸ **2 Tbsp hummus**

Calories: 67 kcal
Total Fat: 3 g
Saturated Fat: 0.5 g
Total Carbohydrate: 8 g
Protein: 3 g
Sodium: 121 mg
Fiber: 2 g

NUTRIENT INTAKE:

45% carbs
17% protein
38% fat

DINNER

▸ Mushroom and Zucchini Pizza

SERVES: 1

Tortillas make a great, extra-thin pizza crust and keeps the calories in this recipe under control.

1 whole wheat flour tortilla
1 tsp olive oil
1 clove garlic, finely chopped
2 Tbsp grated Parmesan cheese
2 Tbsp shredded part-skim mozzarella cheese
½ cup thinly sliced zucchini
½ cup thinly sliced mushrooms
¼ tsp dried oregano

Preheat oven to 425°F.

1. Place tortilla on a baking sheet lined with parchment paper.
2. Brush tortilla with olive oil and sprinkle with garlic, followed by cheeses. Then top with zucchini and mushrooms and sprinkle with oregano.
3. Bake for 10 minutes, until edges are crispy.

Calories: 288 kcal
Total Fat: 13 g
Saturated Fat: 4 g
Total Carbohydrate: 27 g
Protein: 13.5 g
Sodium: 406 mg
Fiber: 3 g

NUTRIENT INTAKE:

38% carbs
19% protein
43% fat

SNACK 4 (OPTIONAL)

- **1 cup air-popped popcorn**

Calories: 31 kcal
Total Fat: 0 g
Saturated Fat: 0 g
Total Carbohydrate: 6 g
Protein: 1 g
Sodium: 1 mg
Fiber: 1 g

NUTRIENT INTAKE:

77% carbs
13% protein
10% fat

NUTRITION FOR THE DAY

Calories: 1215 kcal
Total Fat: 35 g
Saturated Fat: 10 g
Total Carbohydrate: 152 g
Protein: 86 g
Sodium: 2042 mg
Fiber: 28 g

NUTRIENT INTAKE:

53% carbs
23% protein
24% fat

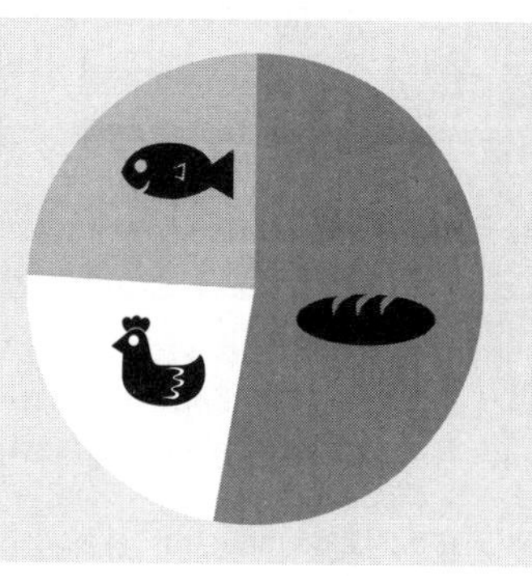

BREAKFAST

- **1 egg + 2 egg whites, scrambled with ½ cup chopped baby spinach and 2 Tbsp crumbled low fat feta**
- **1 slice whole wheat bread, toasted**

Calories: 242 kcal
Total Fat: 10 g
Saturated Fat: 4 g
Total Carbohydrate: 741 g
Protein: 23 g
Sodium: 741 mg
Fiber: 3 g

NUTRIENT INTAKE:

26% carbs
37% protein
37% fat

SNACK 1

- **6 oz nonfat fruit or vanilla yogurt**

Calories: 130 kcal
Total Fat: 0 g
Saturated Fat: 0 g
Total Carbohydrate: 26 g
Protein: 6 g
Sodium: 105 mg
Fiber: 2 g

NUTRIENT INTAKE:

81% carbs
19% protein
0% fat

LUNCH

- **Turkey Sandwich**
  1 whole wheat English muffin, toasted
  3 oz low sodium turkey breast
  3 slices tomato
  2 tsp Dijon mustard

- **1½ cups mixed greens with 1 Tbsp low fat vinaigrette salad dressing**

Calories: 238 kcal
Total Fat: 3.5 g
Saturated Fat: 0 g
Total Carbohydrate: 31 g
Protein: 23 g
Sodium: 801 mg
Fiber: 3 g

NUTRIENT INTAKE:

50% carbs
37% protein
13% fat

SNACK 2

- 1 medium banana

Calories: 105 kcal
Total Fat: 0 g
Saturated Fat: 0 g
Total Carbohydrate: 27 g
Protein: 1 g
Sodium: 1 mg
Fiber: 3 g

NUTRIENT INTAKE:

92% carbs
4% protein
4% fat

SNACK 3

- 1 medium apple
- 1 Tbsp natural peanut butter

Calories: 177 kcal
Total Fat: 8 g
Saturated Fat: 1 g
Total Carbohydrate: 22 g
Protein: 4 g
Sodium: 61 mg
Fiber: 4 g

NUTRIENT INTAKE:

49% carbs
10% protein
41% fat

DINNER

- 1 cup steamed broccoli
- Popcorn Shrimp with Spicy Dipping Sauce

QUICK OPTION MEAL to popcorn shrimp < < < < < < < < <

Green Salad with Shrimp

2 cups mixed greens
½ cup sliced cucumber
¼ cup sliced red onion
½ cup sliced carrots
4 oz cooked shrimp (grilled or roasted)
1 Tbsp sunflower seeds
1 Tbsp balsamic vinegar
2 tsp extra-virgin olive oil

Total Calories: 319 kcal
Total Fat: 15 g
Saturated Fat: 2 g
Total Carbohydrate: 19 g
Protein: 28 g
Sodium: 327 mg
Fiber: 6 g

NUTRIENT INTAKE

23% carbs
35% protein
42% fat

Popcorn Shrimp with Spicy Dipping Sauce

SERVES: 4

Shrimp:

½ cup all-purpose flour
½ tsp kosher salt
¼ tsp black pepper
¼ tsp Old Bay seasoning
2 egg whites
1 Tbsp water
½ cup cornmeal
½ cup panko bread crumbs
1 Tbsp canola oil
Nonstick cooking spray
1 pound large raw shrimp, peeled and deveined

Dipping Sauce:

2 Tbsp nonfat Greek yogurt
2 Tbsp light mayonnaise
2 Tbsp ketchup
1 tsp chili sauce (such as Sriracha)
1 Tbsp freshly squeezed lemon juice

Preheat oven to 400°F

1. Set up a breading station with 3 shallow bowls: place flour, salt, pepper and Old Bay in one bowl; whisk egg whites with 1 Tbsp water in a separate bowl and in the final bowl, combine cornmeal and panko bread crumbs.
2. Toss shrimp in flour, shake off excess and transfer to egg whites and then to cornmeal mixture. Set breaded shrimp aside on a plate.
3. Brush a baking sheet with canola oil. Place shrimp on sheet and spray with nonstick spray and place in oven for about 5 to 6 minutes or until golden and crisp.

For extra crispy shrimp, turn on the broiler for 1 or 2 minutes at the end of cooking (watch carefully to make sure they don't burn!)

Total Calories: 331 kcal
Total Fat: 9 g
Saturated Fat: 1 g
Total Carbohydrate: 34 g
Protein: 31 g
Sodium: 590 mg
Fiber: 7 g

NUTRIENT INTAKE

40% carbs
36% protein
24% fat

SNACK 4 (OPTIONAL)

- ½ cup frozen grapes

Total Calories: 55 kcal
Total Fat: 0 g
Saturated Fat: 0 g
Total Carbohydrate: 14 g
Protein: 1 g
Sodium: 2 mg
Fiber: 1 g

NUTRIENT INTAKE:

94% carbs
4% protein
2% fat

NUTRITION FOR THE DAY

Total Calories: 1174 kcal
Total Fat: 31 g
Saturated Fat: 7 g
Total Carbohydrate: 144 g
Protein: 88 g
Sodium: 2185 mg
Fiber: 21 g

NUTRIENT INTAKE:

62% carbs
21% protein
17% fat

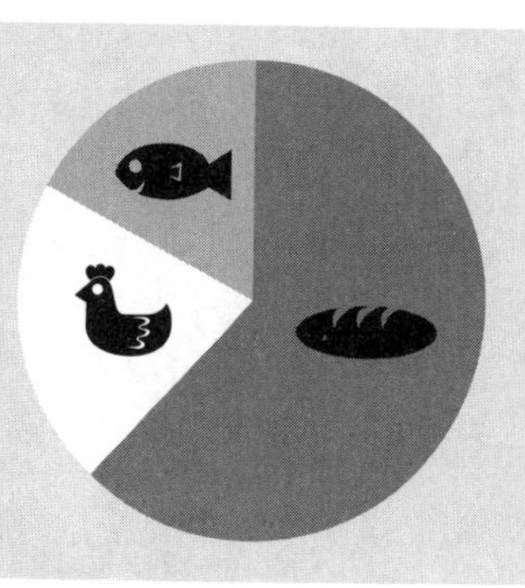

BREAKFAST

▸ Fruit and almond parfait

¾ cup sliced strawberries
½ cup orange segments
½ cup nonfat Greek yogurt
2 Tbsp sliced almonds

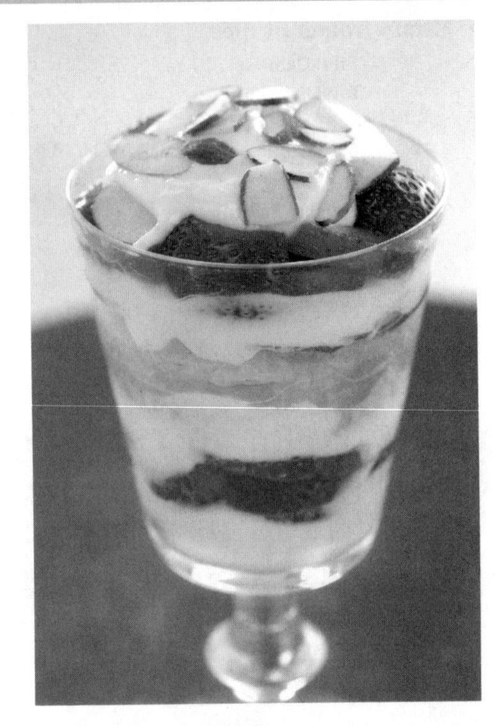

Calories: 212 kcal
Total Fat: 6 g
Saturated Fat: 0.5 g
Total Carbohydrate: 28 g
Protein: 14 g
Sodium: 44 mg
Fiber: 6 g

NUTRIENT INTAKE:

56% carbs
19% protein
25% fat

SNACK 1

▸ 1 hard-boiled egg

Calories: 78 kcal
Total Fat: 5 g
Saturated Fat: 1.5 g
Total Carbohydrate: 1 g
Protein: 6 g
Sodium: 62 mg
Fiber: 0 g

NUTRIENT INTAKE:

3% carbs
33% protein
64% fat

LUNCH

- **Chef's Salad**

2 cups chopped lettuce
½ cup chopped tomato
½ cup sliced cucumber
2 oz low sodium turkey breast
2 Tbsp shredded low fat cheddar cheese
2 tsp olive oil and 2 tsp white wine vinegar

Calories: 195 kcal
Total Fat: 11 g
Saturated Fat: 2 g
Total Carbohydrate: 7 g
Protein: 19 g
Sodium: 501 mg
Fiber: 2 g

NUTRIENT INTAKE:

13% carbs
37% protein
50% fat

SNACK 2

- **½ red bell pepper, sliced**
- **2 Tbsp hummus**

Calories: 62 kcal
Total Fat: 3 g
Saturated Fat: 0 g
Total Carbohydrate: 8 g
Protein: 3 g
Sodium: 107 mg
Fiber: 3 g

NUTRIENT INTAKE:

45% carbs
17% protein
38% fat

SNACK 3

- **1 granola bar (Kashi)**

Calories: 130 kcal
Total Fat: 5 g
Saturated Fat: 0.5 g
Total Carbohydrate: 20 g
Protein: 5 g
Sodium: 90 mg
Fiber: 4 g

NUTRIENT INTAKE:

55% carbs
14% protein
31% fat

DINNER

- 1 cup steamed spinach
- Spaghetti and meatballs

Spaghetti and Meatballs

SERVES: 4

Leftover sauce and meatballs freeze beautifully. Make the whole recipe so you can use the leftovers another time.

Canned tomatoes sometimes need something to bring out their flavor—a small pinch of sugar will do the trick!

1 Tbsp olive oil
1 cup diced onion
2 cloves garlic, minced
¼ tsp kosher salt
⅛ tsp black pepper
2 Tbsp tomato paste
28 oz can diced tomatoes—more lycopene in canned
¼ cup fresh basil, chopped

1 lb ground turkey breast
¼ cup minced onion
1 clove garlic, minced
2 tsp dried oregano
¼ cup seasoned bread crumbs
1 egg, lightly beaten
¼ tsp kosher salt
¼ tsp black pepper

8 oz whole grain pasta (such as Barilla PLUS)

For the sauce:
Heat oil in a medium saucepan; add onion and garlic and cook for 7 to 10 minutes. Season with salt and pepper. Add tomato paste, diced tomatoes, and basil. Reduce heat and simmer for 20 minutes.

For the meatballs:
Preheat oven to 375°F. In a bowl combine turkey, onion, garlic, oregano, bread crumbs, egg, salt and pepper. Mix gently to combine and form into meatballs. Transfer to a baking sheet lined with parchment paper and bake for 30 minutes. When meatballs are cooked, add them to pot with sauce.

Cook pasta according to package directions, drain. Serve pasta with meatballs and sauce.

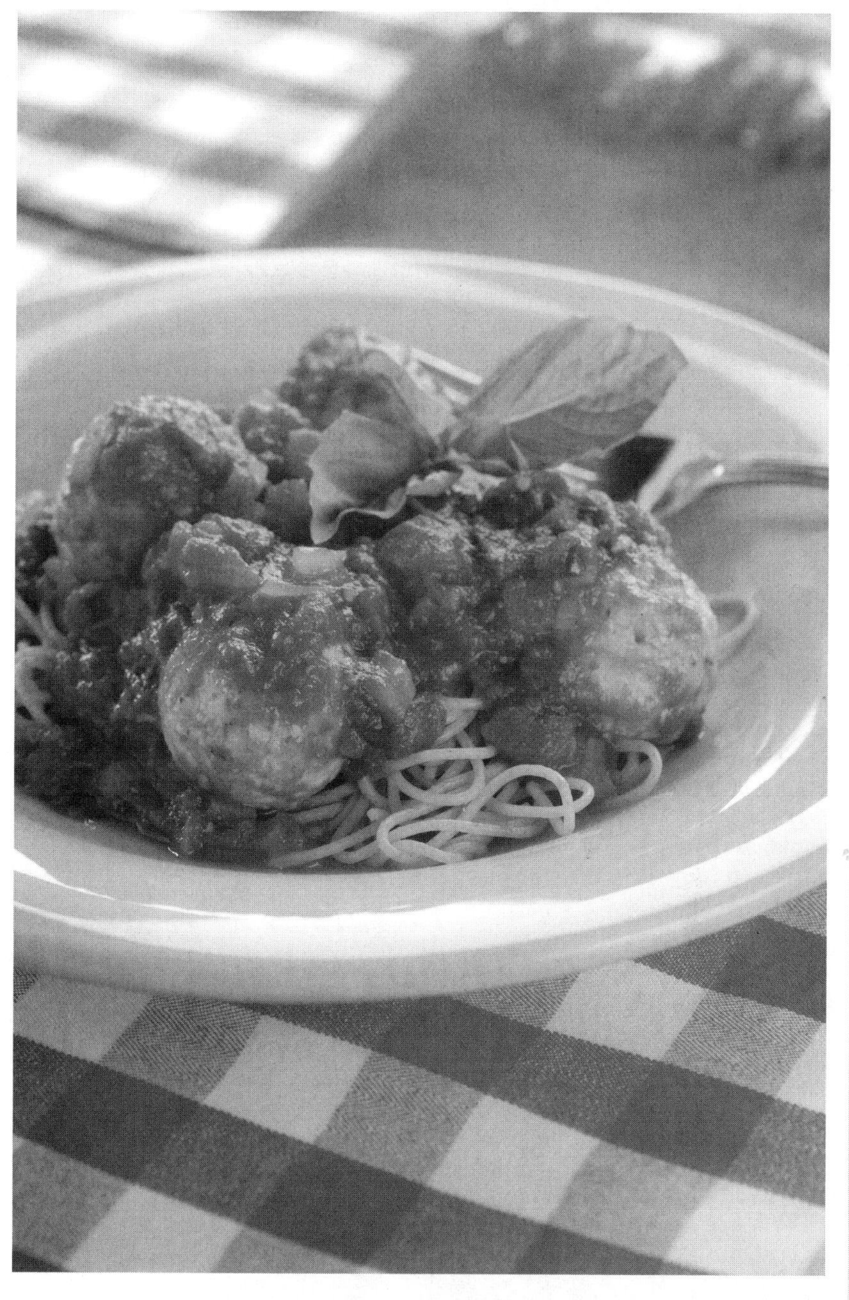

Tomatoes that are canned have more lycopene, which is a powerful antioxidant.

Total Calories: 513 kcal
Total Fat: 7 g
Saturated Fat: 1 g
Total Carbohydrate: 71 g
Protein: 47 g
Sodium: 1074 mg
Fiber: 7 g

NUTRIENT INTAKE:

SNACK 4 (OPTIONAL)

► **1 tangerine**

Calories: 45 kcal
Total Fat: 0 g
Saturated Fat: 0 g
Total Carbohydrate: 11 g
Protein: 1 g
Sodium: 2 mg
Fiber: 2 g

NUTRIENT INTAKE:

90% carbs
5% protein
5% fat

NUTRITION FOR THE DAY

Calories: 1234 kcal
Total Fat: 38 g
Saturated Fat: 6 g
Total Carbohydrate: 145 g
Protein: 95 g
Sodium: 1880 mg
Fiber: 23 g

NUTRIENT INTAKE:

45% carbs
23% protein
32% fat

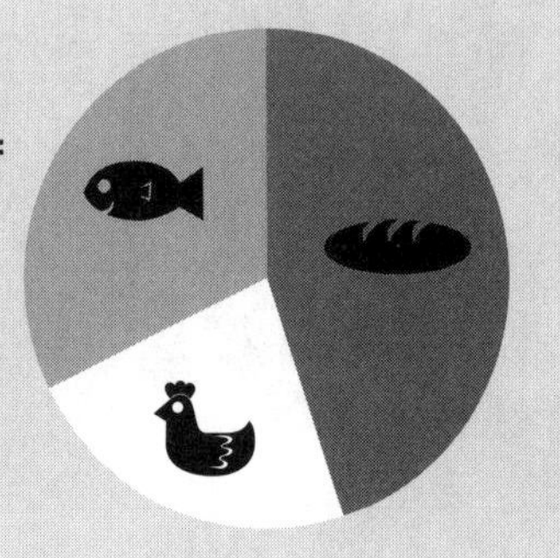

BREAKFAST

- **1 cup cooked oatmeal, topped with ½ tsp cinnamon, 1 tsp honey, and 1 Tbsp raisins**

Whole grain oatmeal contains soluble fiber, which helps lower cholesterol

Total Calories: 199 kcal
Total Fat: 2 g
Saturated Fat: 0 g
Total Carbohydrate: 39 g
Protein: 6 g
Sodium: 4 mg
Fiber: 5 g

NUTRIENT INTAKE:
77% carbs
13% protein
10% fat

SNACK 1

- **½ cup nonfat cottage cheese**
- **½ cup blueberries**

Blueberries are an antioxidant with hunger-fighting fiber.

Total Calories: 103 kcal
Total Fat: 0.5 g
Saturated Fat: 0 g
Total Carbohydrate: 12 g
Protein: 13 g
Sodium: 10 mg
Fiber: 2 g

NUTRIENT INTAKE:
45% carbs
50% protein
5% fat

LUNCH

- **Green Salad with Grilled Chicken**

2 cups mixed greens
½ cup sliced cucumber
¼ cup sliced red onion
½ cup sliced carrots
3 oz grilled chicken breast, sliced
1 Tbsp sunflower seeds
1 Tbsp balsamic vinegar
2 tsp extra-virgin olive oil

Total Calories: 343 kcal
Total Fat: 16 g
Saturated Fat: 2.5 g
Total Carbohydrate: 20 g
Protein: 31 g
Sodium: 141 mg
Fiber: 6 g

NUTRIENT INTAKE:
23% carbs
35% protein
42% fat

SNACK 2

- 1 Tbsp natural peanut butter
- 6 whole wheat crackers

Total Calories: 165 kcal
Total Fat: 9.5 g
Saturated Fat: 1 g
Total Carbohydrate: 13 g
Protein: 6 g
Sodium: 200 mg
Fiber: 3 g

NUTRIENT INTAKE:

32% carbs
15% protein
53% fat

SNACK 3

- 1 medium pear

Total Calories: 96 kcal
Total Fat: 0 g
Saturated Fat: 0 g
Total Carbohydrate: 26 g
Protein: 1 g
Sodium: 2 mg
Fiber: 5 g

NUTRIENT INTAKE:

96% carbs
2% protein
2% fat

DINNER

- 4 oz broiled pork chop (prepared with 1 tsp olive oil and 1 tsp grill seasoning)
- 1 cup steamed green beans
- ½ cup cooked quinoa—whole grain, highest in protein

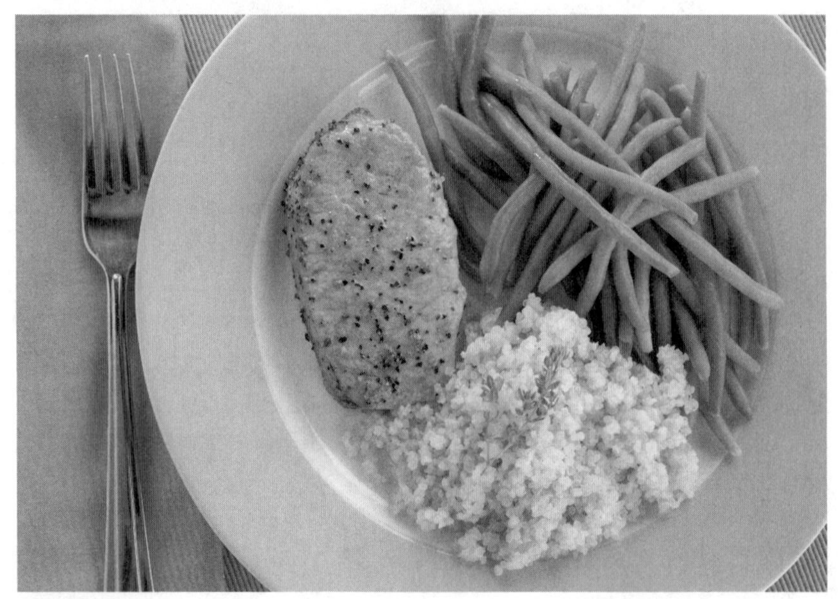

Quinoa, pronounced "keen-wa," is higher in protein than any other whole grain.

Total Calories: 338 kcal
Total Fat: 7 g
Saturated Fat: 2 g
Total Carbohydrate: 29 g
Protein: 40 g
Sodium: 292 mg
Fiber: 7 g

NUTRIENT INTAKE:

35% carbs
47% protein
18% fat

SNACK 4 (OPTIONAL)

- **1 small container sugar-free gelatin**

Total Calories: 10 kcal
Total Fat: 0 g
Saturated Fat: 0 g
Total Carbohydrate: 0 g
Protein: 1 g
Sodium: 45 mg
Fiber: 0 g

NUTRIENT INTAKE:

0% carbs
100% protein
0% fat

NUTRITION FOR THE DAY

Total Calories: 1255 kcal
Total Fat: 36 g
Saturated Fat: 6 g
Total Carbohydrate: 139 g
Protein: 98 g
Sodium: 694 mg
Fiber: 28 g

NUTRIENT INTAKE:

44% carbs
37% protein
19% fat

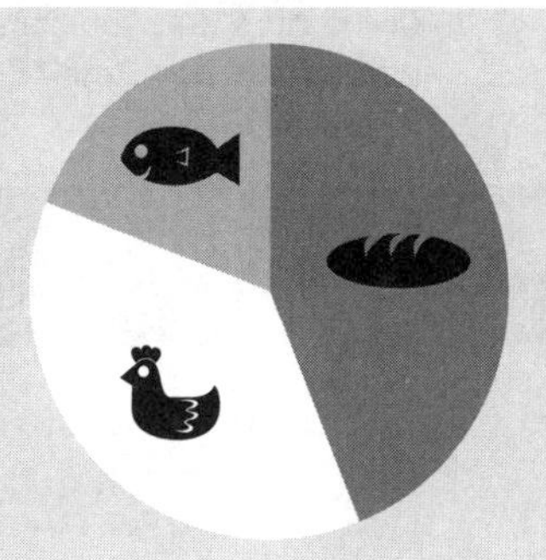

BREAKFAST

- **1 cup whole grain cereal (suggestions: Bran Flakes, Nature's Path Heirloom Flakes)**
- **¾ cup skim milk**
- **½ cup blueberries**

Total Calories: 232 kcal
Total Fat: 1 g
Saturated Fat: 0 g
Total Carbohydrate: 52 g
Protein: 10 g
Sodium: 371 mg
Fiber: 9 g

NUTRIENT INTAKE:

80% carbs
16% protein
4% fat

SNACK 1

▸ Energy Mix

MAKES 6 SERVINGS

¼ cup walnut halves
¼ cup slivered almonds
¼ cup dried cranberries
¼ cup whole grain cereal (such as Kashi Heart to Heart)
2 Tbsp sunflower seeds

1. Combine ingredients in a medium bowl and mix.
2. Divide into 6 equal portions (2 heaping tablespoons per serving) and store in resealable plastic bags.

Walnuts are a plant-based source of healthy omega-3 fats and the antioxidant vitamin E

Total Calories: 146 kcal
Total Fat: 12 g
Saturated Fat: 1 g
Total Carbohydrate: 8 g
Protein: 4 g
Sodium: 10 mg
Fiber: 2 g

NUTRIENT INTAKE:

20% carbs
11% protein
69% fat

LUNCH

▸ Chicken Pita

2 oz deli-sliced chicken breast
3 slices tomato
2 tsp Dijon mustard
½ cup lettuce

Total Calories: 242 kcal
Total Fat: 3 g
Saturated Fat: 1 g
Total Carbohydrate: 34 g
Protein: 20 g
Sodium: 1264 mg
Fiber: 6 g

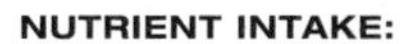

NUTRIENT INTAKE:

55% carbs
33% protein
12% fat

SNACK 2

▸ **1 medium grapefruit**

Total Calories: 82 kcal
Total Fat: 0 g
Saturated Fat: 0 g
Total Carbohydrate: 21 g
Protein: 2 g
Sodium: 0 mg
Fiber: 3 g

NUTRIENT INTAKE:

90% carbs
7% protein
3% fat

SNACK 3

▸ **10 baby carrots**
▸ **1 part-skim mozzarella string cheese**

Calories: 115 kcal
Total Fat: 6 g
Saturated Fat: 3.5 g
Total Carbohydrate: 9 g
Protein: 8 g
Sodium: 298 mg
Fiber: 2 g

NUTRIENT INTAKE:

30% carbs
25% protein
45% fat

DINNER

▸ **Honey-roasted salmon and broccoli**

Honey-Roasted Salmon and Broccoli

SERVES: 1

4 oz wild salmon, skin removed
2 tsp olive oil
1 clove minced garlic
2 tsp honey
2 Tbsp lemon juice
1 cup broccoli florets
Salt and pepper to taste
Lemon wedges

continued

1. Preheat oven to 375°F.
2. Place salmon on one side of a baking sheet lined with parchment paper.
3. In a small bowl, combine oil, garlic, honey, and lemon juice; season with salt and pepper and whisk to combine.
4. Spoon half the honey sauce over the fish and roast for 10 minutes.
5. Add the broccoli to the baking sheet, drizzle with remaining sauce and return to the oven for an additional 7 minutes. Serve with lemon wedges.

Total Calories: 372 kcal
Total Fat: 18 g
Saturated Fat: 3 g
Total Carbohydrate: 21 g
Protein: 34 g
Sodium: 97 mg
Fiber: 3 g

NUTRIENT INTAKE:

22% carbs

36% protein

42% fat

SNACK 4 (OPTIONAL)

▸ **1 cup air-popped popcorn**

Total Calories: 31 kcal
Total Fat: 0 g
Saturated Fat: 0 g
Total Carbohydrate: 6 g
Protein: 1 g
Sodium: 1 mg
Fiber: 1 g

NUTRIENT INTAKE:

77% carbs

13% protein

10% fat

NUTRITION FOR THE DAY

Total Calories: 1220 kcal
Total Fat: 41 g
Saturated Fat: 9 g
Total Carbohydrate: 151 g
Protein: 79 g
Sodium: 2040 mg
Fiber: 26 g

NUTRIENT INTAKE:

53% carbs

20% protein

26% fat

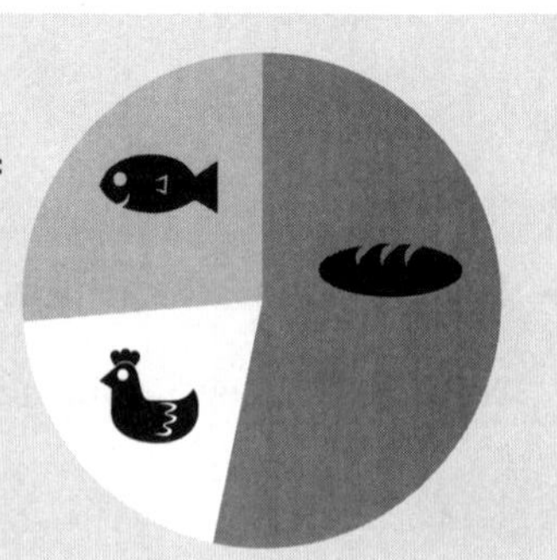

BREAKFAST

- **¾ cup nonfat cottage cheese**
- **½ cup chopped pineapple**
- **2 Tbsp slivered almonds**

Total Calories: 215 kcal
Total Fat: 7.5 g
Saturated Fat: 1 g
Total Carbohydrate: 14 g
Protein: 22 g
Sodium: 15 mg
Fiber: 3 g

NUTRIENT INTAKE:

27% carbs
42% protein
31% fat

SNACK 1

- **½ cup shelled edamame**

Edamame are soybeans and packed with protein. Find them in the freezer section of your grocery store.

Total Calories: 90 kcal
Total Fat: 4 g
Saturated Fat: 1 g
Total Carbohydrate: 7 g
Protein: 8 g
Sodium: 7.5 mg
Fiber: 2 g

NUTRIENT INTAKE:

30% carbs
33% protein
37% fat

LUNCH

- **Quinoa Salad**

1 cup cooked quinoa
½ cup diced cucumber
¼ cup canned chickpeas, rinsed and drained
½ cup grape tomatoes, halved
2 Tbsp light vinaigrette salad dressing

When choosing light vinaigrette salad dressings, go with one that's 60 calories or fewer per serving.

Total Calories: 350 kcal
Total Fat: 8 g
Saturated Fat: 1 g
Total Carbohydrate: 59 g
Protein: 12 g
Sodium: 665 mg
Fiber: 9 g

NUTRIENT INTAKE:

66% carbs
13% protein
21% fat

SNACK 2

- 1 granola bar (Kashi)

Total Calories: 130 kcal
Total Fat: 5 g
Saturated Fat: 0.5 g
Total Carbohydrate: 20 g
Protein: 5 g
Sodium: 90 mg
Fiber: 4 g

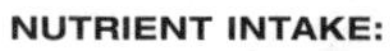

NUTRIENT INTAKE:

55% carbs
14% protein
31% fat

SNACK 3

- 1 cup chopped cantaloupe—high in beta-carotene

Total Calories: 53 kcal
Total Fat: 0 g
Saturated Fat: 0 g
Total Carbohydrate: 13 g
Protein: 1 g
Sodium: 25 mg
Fiber: 1 g

NUTRIENT INTAKE:

86% carbs
9% protein
5% fat

Cantaloupes are high in beta-carotene

DINNER

- 4 oz grilled chicken breast
- 1½ cups cauliflower roasted with 2 tsp olive oil (roast at 400ºF for 15 to 20 minutes), salt and pepper
- 1½ cups mixed greens topped with 1 tsp olive oil and lemon juice

Cauliflower is packed with antioxidants and nutrients.

Total Calories: 365 kcal
Total Fat: 18 g
Saturated Fat: 3 g
Total Carbohydrate: 13 g
Protein: 39 g
Sodium: 149 mg
Fiber: 6 g

NUTRIENT INTAKE:

14% carbs
43% protein
43% fat

SNACK 4 (OPTIONAL)

▸ **1 medium tangerine**

Total Calories: 45 kcal
Total Fat: 0 g
Saturated Fat: 0 g
Total Carbohydrate: 11 g
Protein: 1 g
Sodium: 2 mg
Fiber: 2 g

NUTRIENT INTAKE:

90% carbs
5% protein
5% fat

NUTRITION FOR THE DAY

Total Calories: 1247 kcal
Total Fat: 43 g
Saturated Fat: 6 g
Total Carbohydrate: 137 g
Protein: 88 g
Sodium: 955 mg
Fiber: 27 g

NUTRIENT INTAKE:

52% carbs
23% protein
25% fat

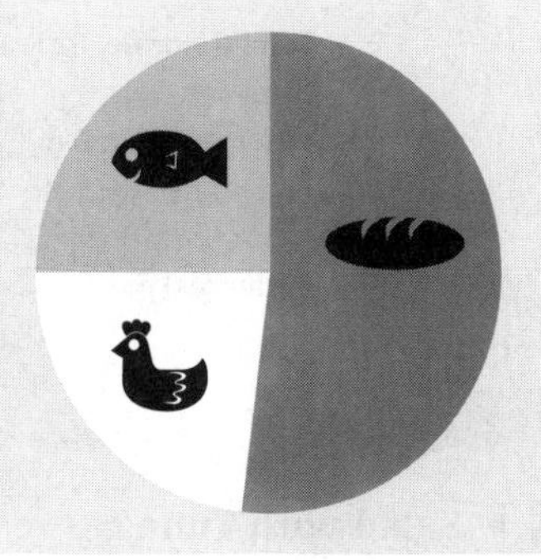

BREAKFAST

- **2 hard-boiled eggs**
- **1 granola bar (Kashi)**

Total Calories: 285 kcal
Total Fat: 15.5 g
Saturated Fat: 4 g
Total Carbohydrate: 21 g
Protein: 18 g
Sodium: 214 mg
Fiber: 4 g

NUTRIENT INTAKE:

29% carbs
24% protein
47% fat

SNACK 1

- **1 medium grapefruit**

Total Calories: 82 kcal
Total Fat: 0 g
Saturated Fat: 0 g
Total Carbohydrate: 21 g
Protein: 2 g
Sodium: 0 mg
Fiber: 3 g

NUTRIENT INTAKE:

90% carbs
7% protein
3% fat

LUNCH

- **Salad with Tuna**

3 oz canned tuna, in water
1 cup grape tomatoes, halved
½ cup frozen green peas, thawed
2 cups mixed greens
2 Tbsp light vinaigrette salad dressing

Total Calories: 237 kcal
Total Fat: 6 g
Saturated Fat: 0.5 g
Total Carbohydrate: 22 g
Protein: 26 g
Sodium: 960 mg
Fiber: 7 g

NUTRIENT INTAKE:

35% carbs
43% protein
22% fat

SNACK 2

▸ **1 medium pear**

Total Calories: 96 kcal
Total Fat: 0 g
Saturated Fat: 0 g
Total Carbohydrate: 39 g
Protein: 7 g
Sodium: 202 mg
Fiber: 8 g

NUTRIENT INTAKE:

96% carbs
2% protein
2% fat

SNACK 3

▸ **Energy mix (see recipe on page 68)**

Total Calories: 146 kcal
Total Fat: 12 g
Saturated Fat: 1 g
Total Carbohydrate: 8 g
Protein: 4 g
Sodium: 10 mg
Fiber: 2 g

NUTRIENT INTAKE:

20% carbs
11% protein
69% fat

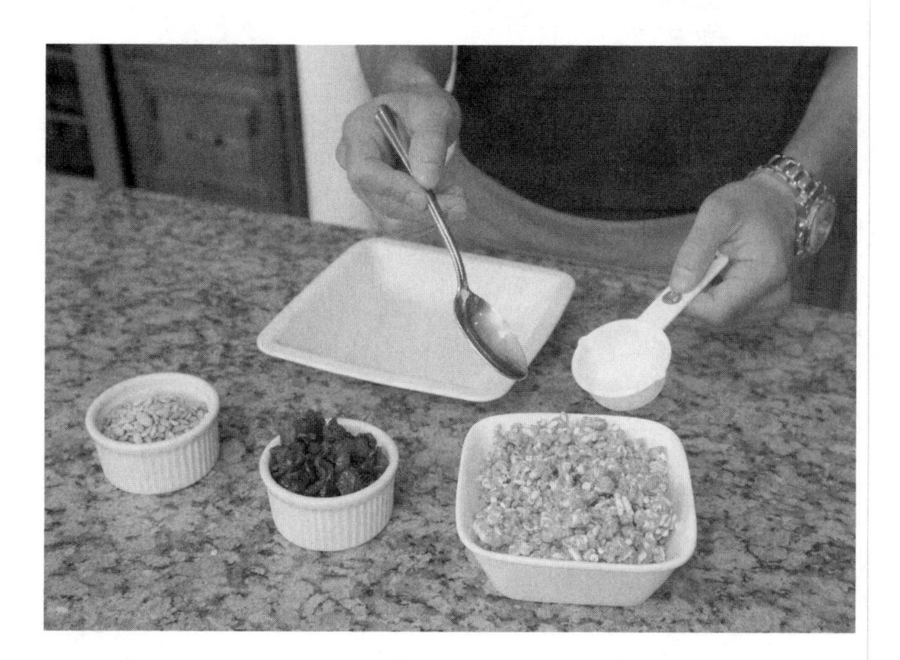

DINNER

- Beef stir-fry (see recipe on page 51)

NUTRITION INFORMATION FOR THE MEAL:

Total Calories: 333 kcal
Total Fat: 11 g
Saturated Fat: 3 g
Total Carbohydrate: 30 g
Protein: 31 g
Sodium: 865 mg
Fiber: 4 g

NUTRIENT INTAKE:

35% carbs
36% protein
29% fat

DESSERT

- ½ cup nonfat vanilla frozen yogurt
- ½ cup chopped pineapple

Total Calories: 127 kcal
Total Fat: 0 g
Saturated Fat: 0 g
Total Carbohydrate: 29 g
Protein: 3 g
Sodium: 46 mg
Fiber: 1 g

NUTRIENT INTAKE:

89% carbs
11% protein
0% fat

NUTRITION FOR THE DAY

Total Calories: 1161 kcal
Total Fat: 33 g
Saturated Fat: 7 g
Total Carbohydrate: 148 g
Protein: 80 g
Sodium: 2287 mg
Fiber: 25 g

NUTRIENT INTAKE:

56% carbs
19% protein
25% fat

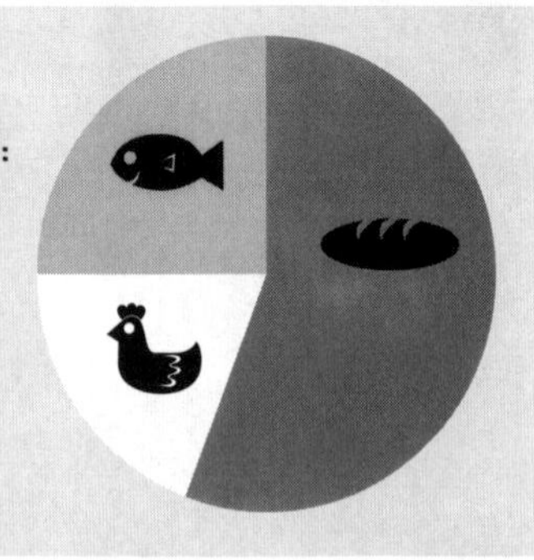

BREAKFAST

- **1 slice whole wheat bread, toasted**
- **1 Tbsp natural peanut butter**
- **1 cup chopped cantaloupe**

Total Calories: 269 kcal
Total Fat: 10 g
Saturated Fat: 2 g
Total Carbohydrate: 36 g
Protein: 9 g
Sodium: 236 mg
Fiber: 5 g

NUTRIENT INTAKE:

53% carbs
14% protein
33% fat

SNACK 1

- **½ cup shelled edamame**

Total Calories: 90 kcal
Total Fat: 4 g
Saturated Fat: 1 g
Total Carbohydrate: 7 g
Protein: 8 g
Sodium: 7.5 mg
Fiber: 2 g

NUTRIENT INTAKE:

30% carbs
33% protein
37% fat

LUNCH

- **1½ cups low sodium lentil soup (Amy's)**
- **15 medium baby carrots**

Total Calories: 278 kcal
Total Fat: 6 g
Saturated Fat: 1 g
Total Carbohydrate: 47 g
Protein: 11 g
Sodium: 627 mg
Fiber: 12 g

NUTRIENT INTAKE:

65% carbs
16% protein
19% fat

SNACK 2

- **½ cup nonfat cottage cheese**
- **½ cup blueberries**

Total Calories: 103 kcal
Total Fat: 0.5 g
Saturated Fat: 0 g
Total Carbohydrate: 12 g
Protein: 13 g
Sodium: 10 mg
Fiber: 2 g

NUTRIENT INTAKE:

45% carbs
50% protein
5% fat

SNACK 3

▸ **1 part-skim mozzarella string cheese**

Total Calories: 80 kcal
Total Fat: 6 g
Saturated Fat: 3.5 g
Total Carbohydrate: 1 g
Protein: 7 g
Sodium: 230 mg
Fiber: 2 g

NUTRIENT INTAKE:

5% carbs
33% protein
62% fat

DINNER

▸ **Quinoa stuffed peppers**

Quinoa Stuffed Peppers

SERVES: 1

2 red bell peppers
2 tsp olive oil
1 cup diced eggplant
1 cup sliced mushrooms
½ cup chopped red onion
Pinch kosher salt
½ tsp black pepper
2 cloves garlic, minced
2 tsp fresh thyme
1 cup low sodium vegetable or chicken broth, divided
1 Tbsp tomato paste
2 Tbsp grated Parmesan or pecorino Romano cheese
½ cup cooked quinoa

1. Lay peppers on their sides and trim the bottom to create a flat surface.
2. Cut tops off peppers and scoop out seeds, set aside.
3. Heat oil in a skillet, add eggplant, mushrooms, and onion; season with salt and pepper and sauté for 3 to 5 minutes until tender.
4. Add garlic, thyme, ½ cup vegetable broth, and tomato paste and continue to cook for an additional 2 minutes.
5. Turn off heat and mix in cheese and quinoa.
6. Fill each pepper with ½ of the quinoa mixture and transfer to a baking dish.
7. Pour remaining ½ cup broth in the bottom of the baking dish. Cover with aluminum foil and bake for 15 minutes, remove foil and bake for 10 more minutes.

Total Calories: 427 kcal
Total Fat: 16 g
Saturated Fat: 4 g
Total Carbohydrate: 58 g
Protein: 20 g
Sodium: 255 mg
Fiber: 13 g

NUTRIENT INTAKE:

51% carbs
18% protein
31% fat

SNACK 4 (OPTIONAL)

▸ **1 small container sugar-free gelatin**

Total Calories: 10 kcal
Total Fat: 0 g
Saturated Fat: 0 g
Total Carbohydrate: 0 g
Protein: 1 g
Sodium: 45 mg
Fiber: 0 g

NUTRIENT INTAKE:

0% carbs

100% protein

0% fat

NUTRITION FOR THE DAY

Total Calories: 1256 kcal
Total Fat: 42.5 g
Saturated Fat: 11 g
Total Carbohydrate: 161 g
Protein: 69 g
Sodium: 1410 mg
Fiber: 34 g

NUTRIENT INTAKE:

36% carbs

38% protein

26% fat

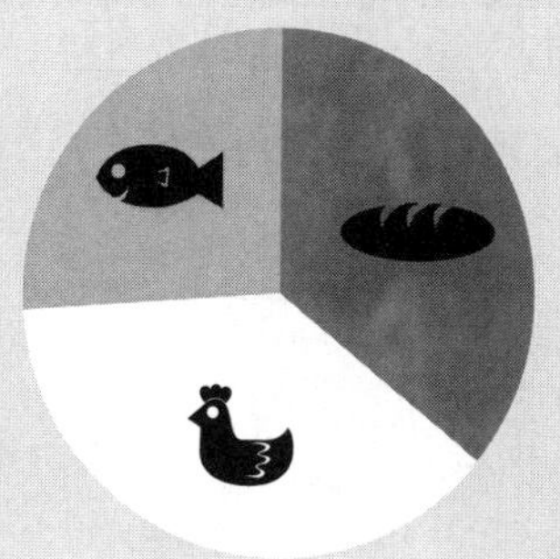

BREAKFAST

▸ **Blueberry muffins**

QUICK OPTION MEAL to blueberry muffins < < < < < < < < < <

1 cup cooked oatmeal, topped with ½ tsp cinnamon, 1 tsp honey, and ¼ cup blueberries

Total Calories: 200 kcal
Total Fat: 2.5 g
Saturated Fat: 0 g
Total Carbohydrate: 39 g
Protein: 7 g
Sodium: 4 mg
Fiber: 6 g

NUTRIENT INTAKE:

75% carbs
14% protein
11% fat

Blueberry Muffins

MAKES 10 MUFFINS

Freeze leftover muffins in a plastic bag—microwave for 15 to 30 seconds to reheat.

1¼ cups all purpose flour
¼ cup sugar
½ tsp baking powder
1 tsp baking soda
½ tsp salt
¼ tsp ground cinnamon

¼ cup maple syrup
¼ cup unsweetened applesauce
¼ cup canola oil
½ cup low fat buttermilk
½ tsp lemon zest
1 large egg
1 tsp vanilla

1 cup blueberries

1. Preheat oven to 375°F.
2. Line a muffin pan with paper liners.
3. In a large bowl sift together flour, sugar, baking powder, baking soda, salt, and cinnamon.
4. In a separate bowl whisk together syrup, applesauce, oil, buttermilk, lemon zest, egg, and vanilla.
5. Add wet ingredients to dry and fold well to combine. Gently fold in blueberries. Using a ⅓ cup measure, scoop batter into muffin pans and bake for 20 minutes until puffed and golden.

Replacing some of the oil with unsweetened applesauce cuts down the fat and calories.

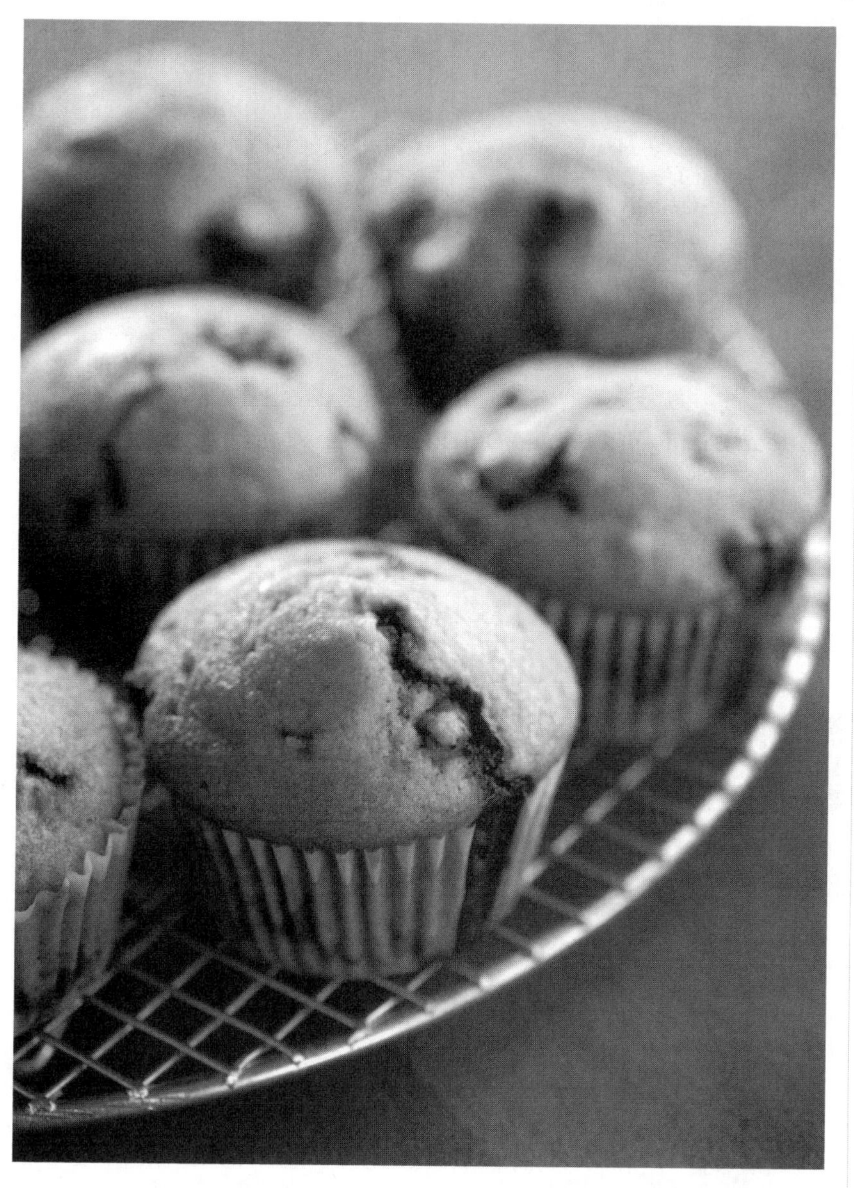

Total Calories: 176 kcal
Total Fat: 6 g
Saturated Fat: 0.5 g
Total Carbohydrate: 28 g
Protein: 3 g
Sodium: 287 mg
Fiber: 1 g

NUTRIENT INTAKE:

62% carbs

6% protein

32% fat

SNACK 1

▸ **1 medium pear**

Total Calories: 96 kcal
Total Fat: 0 g
Saturated Fat: 0 g
Total Carbohydrate: 39 g
Protein: 7 g
Sodium: 202 mg
Fiber: 8 g

NUTRIENT INTAKE:

96% carbs
2% protein
2% fat

LUNCH

▸ **Green Salad with Grilled Chicken**

2 cups mixed greens
½ cup sliced cucumber
¼ cup sliced red onion
½ cup sliced carrots
3 oz grilled chicken breast, sliced
1 Tbsp sunflower seeds
1 Tbsp balsamic vinegar
2 tsp extra-virgin olive oil

Sunflower seeds are packed with vitamins and contain healthy fats.

Total Calories: 347 kcal
Total Fat: 16 g
Saturated Fat: 2.5 g
Total Carbohydrate: 20 g
Protein: 31 g
Sodium: 136 mg
Fiber: 6 g

NUTRIENT INTAKE:

23% carbs
35% protein
42% fat

SNACK 2

▸ **Energy mix (see recipe on page 68)**

Total Calories: 146 kcal
Total Fat: 12 g
Saturated Fat: 1 g
Total Carbohydrate: 8 g
Protein: 4 g
Sodium: 10 mg
Fiber: 2 g

NUTRIENT INTAKE:

20% carbs
11% protein
69% fat

SNACK 3

- 1 cup air-popped popcorn

Total Calories: 31 kcal
Total Fat: 0 g
Saturated Fat: 0 g
Total Carbohydrate: 6 g
Protein: 1 g
Sodium: 1 mg
Fiber: 1 g

NUTRIENT INTAKE:

81% carbs
9% protein
10% fat

DINNER

- Roasted turkey breast
- 1 small baked potato topped with 1 Tbsp nonfat plain yogurt
- ½ cup green peas

Roasted Turkey Breast

SERVES: 4

Aromatic veggies take the place of a baking rack in this recipe. Leftovers are perfect for sandwiches—with a lot less sodium than cold cuts.

2 Tbsp honey
¾ cup low sodium chicken or vegetable broth
2 carrots
1 onion, quartered
1 head garlic, cut in half
1 tsp olive oil
2 to 2.5 lb turkey breast (bone-in, skin on)
Salt and pepper

1. Preheat oven to 375°F.
2. Combine honey and broth, whisk well—set aside.
3. Place carrots, onion, and garlic in the bottom of a baking dish or sheet pan and place turkey breast on top; season well with salt and pepper.
4. Roast turkey for 45 to 60 minutes or until the internal temperature reaches 160°F, basting with a few tablespoons of broth mixture every 15 minutes (you won't need to use all the broth).
5. Remove from oven and allow to rest for at least 15 minutes before removing skin and slicing.

NUTRITION INFORMATION FOR THE MEAL:

Total Calories: 459 kcal
Total Fat: 12.5 g
Saturated Fat: 3.5 g
Total Carbohydrate: 39 g
Protein: 45 g
Sodium: 453 mg
Fiber: 7 g

NUTRIENT INTAKE:

35% carbs
40% protein
25% fat

SNACK 4 (OPTIONAL)

▸ **1 medium tangerine**

Total Calories: 45 kcal
Total Fat: 0 g
Saturated Fat: 0 g
Total Carbohydrate: 11 g
Protein: 1 g
Sodium: 2 mg
Fiber: 2 g

NUTRIENT INTAKE:

90% carbs
5% protein
5% fat

NUTRITION FOR THE DAY

Total Calories: 1301 kcal
Total Fat: 48 g
Saturated Fat: 8 g
Total Carbohydrate: 138 g
Protein: 85 g
Sodium: 890 mg
Fiber: 24 g

NUTRIENT INTAKE:

58% carbs
15% protein
26% fat

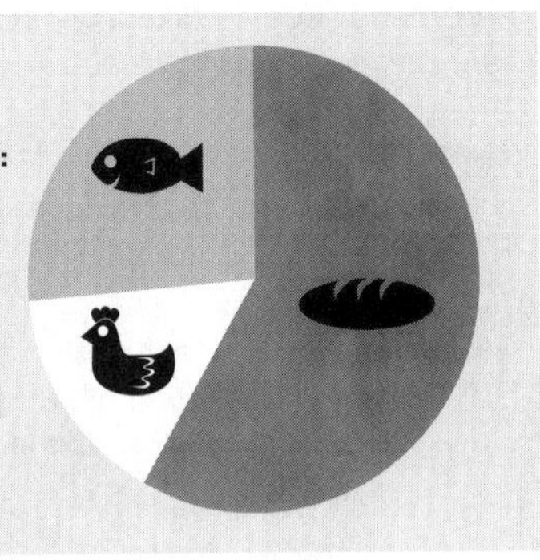

BREAKFAST

- **1 egg + 2 egg whites, scrambled with ½ cup chopped bell pepper and 2 Tbsp grated Parmesan cheese**
- **1 cup skim milk**

Total Calories: 251 kcal
Total Fat: 8.5 g
Saturated Fat: 3.5 g
Total Carbohydrate: 16 g
Protein: 26 g
Sodium: 463 mg
Fiber: 1 g

NUTRIENT INTAKE:

26% carbs
43% protein
31% fat

SNACK 1

- **1 cup chopped cantaloupe**

Total Calories: 55 kcal
Total Fat: 0 g
Saturated Fat: 0 g
Total Carbohydrate: 13 g
Protein: 1 g
Sodium: 26 mg
Fiber: 1 g

NUTRIENT INTAKE:

87% carbs
9% protein
4% fat

LUNCH

- **Turkey Sandwich**

2 slices whole wheat bread, toasted
3 oz roasted turkey breast (from Day 6 dinner)
4 slices, sliced cucumber
1 tsp olive oil and 2 tsp balsamic vinegar

Total Calories: 378 kcal
Total Fat: 12 g
Saturated Fat: 3 g
Total Carbohydrate: 42 g
Protein: 24 g
Sodium: 336 mg
Fiber: 6 g

NUTRIENT INTAKE:

45% carbs
27% protein
28% fat

SNACK 2

▸ **15 baby carrots**

Total Calories: 53 kcal
Total Fat: 0 g
Saturated Fat: 0 g
Total Carbohydrate: 12 g
Protein: 1 g
Sodium: 117 mg
Fiber: 3 g

NUTRIENT INTAKE:

90% carbs
5% protein
5% fat

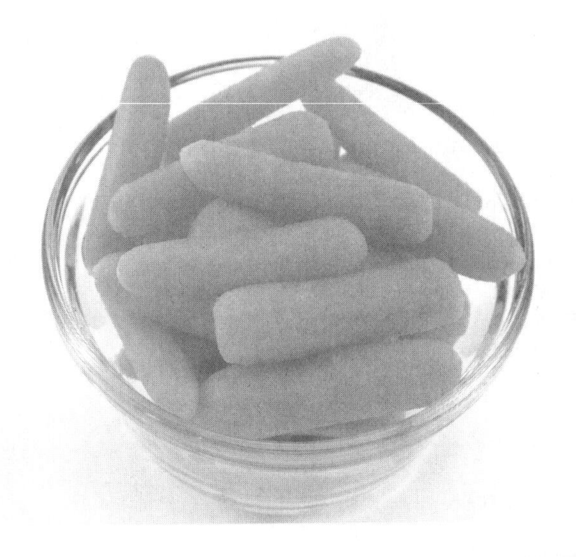

SNACK 3

▸ **½ cup shelled edamame**

Total Calories: 90 kcal
Total Fat: 4 g
Saturated Fat: 1 g
Total Carbohydrate: 7 g
Protein: 8 g
Sodium: 7.5 mg
Fiber: 2 g

NUTRIENT INTAKE:

30% carbs
33% protein
37% fat

DINNER

- 4 oz grilled shrimp in a pita with 1 cup mixed greens
- 1½ cups cauliflower roasted with 2 tsp olive oil, salt and pepper

Total Calories: 412 kcal
Total Fat: 12 g
Saturated Fat: 2 g
Total Carbohydrate: 46 g
Protein: 34 g
Sodium: 653 mg
Fiber: 10 g

NUTRIENT INTAKE:

43% carbs
32% protein
25% fat

SNACK 4 (OPTIONAL)

- ½ cup chopped pineapple

Total Calories: 37 kcal
Total Fat: 0 g
Saturated Fat: 0 g
Total Carbohydrate: 10 g
Protein: 0 g
Sodium: 1 mg
Fiber: 1 g

NUTRIENT INTAKE:

94% carbs
4% protein
2% fat

NUTRITION FOR THE DAY

Total Calories: 1275 kcal
Total Fat: 37 g
Saturated Fat: 9 g
Total Carbohydrate: 146 g
Protein: 95 g
Sodium: 1603 mg
Fiber: 24 g

NUTRIENT INTAKE:

59% carbs
22% protein
19% fat

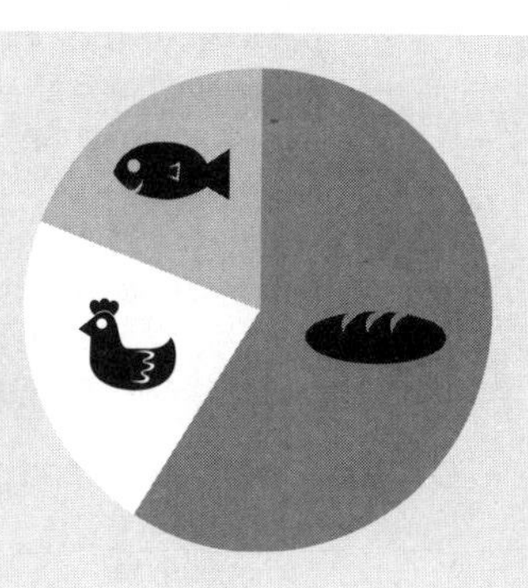

BREAKFAST

▸ **1 cup cooked oatmeal topped with ½ sliced banana* and 1 Tbsp toasted wheat germ (antioxidants, vitamin E, nutty crunch for less fat than nuts)**

**save remaining ½ banana in the fridge for tomorrow's smoothie*

Total Calories: 227 kcal
Total Fat: 3 g
Saturated Fat: 0.5 g
Total Carbohydrate: 42 g
Protein: 9 g
Sodium: 3 mg
Fiber: 7 g

NUTRIENT INTAKE:
72% carbs
15% protein
13% fat

Wheat germ adds a nutty flavor and crunch for fewer calories than nuts. It's also packed with antioxidants and vitamin E.

SNACK 1

▸ **¼ cup cashews**

Total Calories: 197 kcal
Total Fat: 16 g
Saturated Fat: 3 g
Total Carbohydrate: 11 g
Protein: 5 g
Sodium: 6 mg
Fiber: 1 g

NUTRIENT INTAKE:
21% carbs
11% protein
68% fat

LUNCH

▸ **Grilled Chicken Caesar Salad**
2 cups romaine lettuce
½ cup sliced cucumber
¼ cup sliced red onion
4 oz grilled chicken breast, sliced
2 Tbsp light Caesar dressing

Total Calories: 302 kcal
Total Fat: 10 g
Saturated Fat: 2 g
Total Carbohydrate: 13 g
Protein: 38 g
Sodium: 632 mg
Fiber: 3 g

NUTRIENT INTAKE:
17% carbs
52% protein
31% fat

SNACK 2

- ½ cup raspberries

Total Calories: 40 kcal
Total Fat: 0 g
Saturated Fat: 0 g
Total Carbohydrate: 9 g
Protein: 1 g
Sodium: 1 mg
Fiber: 5 g

NUTRIENT INTAKE:

83% carbs
8% protein
9% fat

SNACK 3

- 1 medium apple
- 1 part-skim mozzarella string cheese

Total Calories: 152 kcal
Total Fat: 6 g
Saturated Fat: 3.5 g
Total Carbohydrate: 20 g
Protein: 7 g
Sodium: 221 mg
Fiber: 3 g

NUTRIENT INTAKE:

48% carbs
18% protein
34% fat

DINNER

- Veggie chili

Veggie Chili

SERVES: 8

Make the entire batch and freeze leftovers for another night. Swap zucchini for butternut squash when it's in season.

1 Tbsp olive oil
½ cup chopped red onion
½ cup chopped red bell pepper
1 finely chopped jalapeño pepper (optional)
½ cup chopped celery
½ tsp kosher salt
1 clove minced garlic
1 tsp ground cumin
½ cup vegetable broth or water
1 tsp Worcestershire sauce
1 cup dark beer
2 28 oz cans crushed tomatoes
1 15 oz can tomato sauce

Cooking with a small amount of alcohol provides extra flavor, and most of the calories get cooked out.

continued

Pinch cayenne pepper
2 Tbsp chili powder, or to taste
½ tsp celery salt
2 tsp dried tarragon
1 15 oz can garbanzo beans, rinsed and drained
1 15 oz can red kidney beans, rinsed and drained
1 15 oz can black beans, rinsed and drained
¾ cup frozen corn kernels
1 cup diced zucchini
1 sweet potato, peeled and diced small

Garnish (per person)
1 Tbsp sliced black olives
1 Tbsp nonfat plain Greek yogurt
Chopped scallions
5 baked tortilla chips

1. Heat oil in large pot or Dutch oven over medium heat.
2. Sauté onion, peppers, and celery for 3 to 5 minutes until tender, season with salt.
3. Add garlic and cumin, cook for 1 minute—stirring gently to toast cumin.
4. Stir in vegetable broth, Worcestershire, beer, crushed tomatoes, and tomato sauce.
5. Add cayenne, chili powder, celery salt, and tarragon.
6. Stir in beans; taste to adjust seasoning (add more salt or chili powder, if desired). Bring to a simmer and cook uncovered for 20 minutes, stirring occasionally.
7. Add corn, zucchini, and sweet potato, cook for an additional 30 minutes or until sweet potato is tender. Serve with chips, olives, yogurt, and scallions.

Total Calories: 312 kcal
Total Fat: 5 g
Saturated Fat: 0.5 g
Total Carbohydrate: 56 g
Protein: 13 g
Sodium: 1084 mg
Fiber: 13 g

NUTRIENT INTAKE:

68% carbs
16% protein
14% fat

SNACK 4 (OPTIONAL)

▸ **1 cup air-popped popcorn**

Total Calories: 31 kcal
Total Fat: 0 g
Saturated Fat: 0 g
Total Carbohydrate: 6 g
Protein: 1 g
Sodium: 1 mg
Fiber: 1 g

NUTRIENT INTAKE:

NUTRITION FOR THE DAY

Total Calories: 1252 kcal
Total Fat: 41 g
Saturated Fat: 10 g
Total Carbohydrate: 156 g
Protein: 74 g
Sodium: 1949 mg
Fiber: 32 g

NUTRIENT INTAKE:

55% carbs
19% protein
26% fat

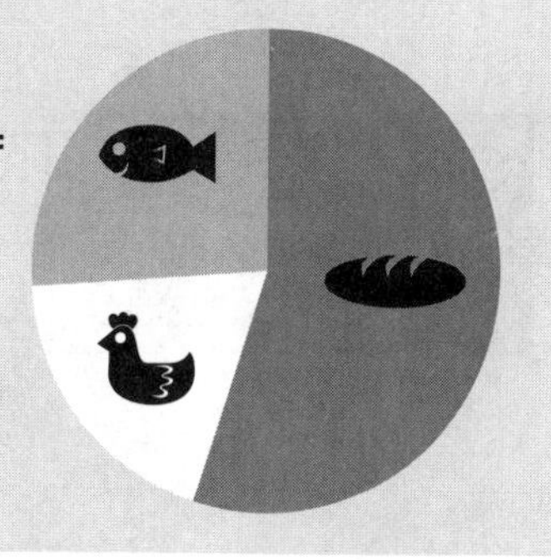

BREAKFAST

▸ Tropical smoothie

SERVES: 1

½ medium banana
½ cup chopped mango
½ cup frozen pineapple chunks
½ cup nonfat plain Greek yogurt
½ cup orange juice
Ice

Place ingredients in a blender and blend until smooth.

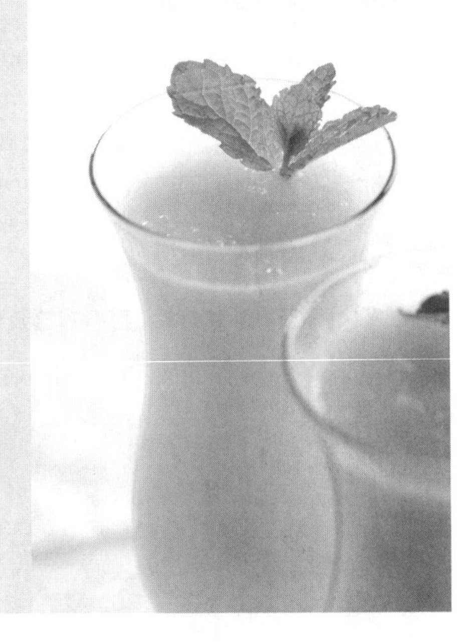

Frozen fruit makes a creamier, frothier smoothie.

Total Calories: 263 kcal
Total Fat: 0.5 g
Saturated Fat: 0 g
Total Carbohydrate: 62 g
Protein: 11 g
Sodium: 88 mg
Fiber: 4 g

NUTRIENT INTAKE:

82% carbs
17% protein
1% fat

SNACK 1

- **10 celery sticks**
- **1 Tbsp almond butter**

Different kinds of nut butters are a great way to get your hunger-fighting healthy fats.

Total Calories: 107 kcal
Total Fat: 9.5 g
Saturated Fat: 1 g
Total Carbohydrate: 5 g
Protein: 3 g
Sodium: 104 mg
Fiber: 1 g

NUTRIENT INTAKE:

16% carbs
9% protein
75% fat

LUNCH

▸ Roast Beef and Swiss Wrap

1 whole wheat tortilla (6 inch)
3 oz low sodium roast beef
1 slice low fat Swiss cheese
2 slices tomato
2 tsp Dijon mustard
½ cup fresh arugula

Total Calories: 338 kcal
Total Fat: 9 g
Saturated Fat: 3 g
Total Carbohydrate: 25 g
Protein: 33 g
Sodium: 546 mg
Fiber: 2 g

NUTRIENT INTAKE:

32% carbs
42% protein
26% fat

SNACK 2

▸ 1 hard-boiled egg

Total Calories: 78 kcal
Total Fat: 5 g
Saturated Fat: 1.5 g
Total Carbohydrate: 1 g
Protein: 6 g
Sodium: 62 mg
Fiber: 0 g

NUTRIENT INTAKE:

3% carbs
35% protein
62% fat

SNACK 3

▸ ¼ cup dried apricots

Dried fruit contains iron and fiber; small portions make an easy on-the-go snack.

Total Calories: 100 kcal
Total Fat: 0 g
Saturated Fat: 0 g
Total Carbohydrate: 26 g
Protein: 7 g
Sodium: 62 mg
Fiber: 3 g

NUTRIENT INTAKE:

96% carbs
4% protein
0% fat

DINNER

- 4 oz broiled pork chop (prepared with 1 tsp olive oil and 1 tsp grill seasoning)
- 2 cups arugula topped with ½ cup chopped tomato and 2 tsp olive oil and lemon juice

Total Calories: 336 kcal
Total Fat: 18.5 g
Saturated Fat: 4.5 g
Total Carbohydrate: 5.5 g
Protein: 36 g
Sodium: 84 mg
Fiber: 4 g

NUTRIENT INTAKE:

7% carbs
43% protein
50% fat

SNACK 4 (OPTIONAL)

- ½ cup pineapple

Total Calories: 37 kcal
Total Fat: 0 g
Saturated Fat: 0 g
Total Carbohydrate: 10 g
Protein: 0 g
Sodium: 1 mg
Fiber: 1 g

NUTRIENT INTAKE:

94% carbs
4% protein
2% fat

NUTRITION FOR THE DAY

Total Calories: 1259 kcal
Total Fat: 43 g
Saturated Fat: 10.5 g
Total Carbohydrate: 134 g
Protein: 91 g
Sodium: 884 mg
Fiber: 18 g

NUTRIENT INTAKE:

47% carbs
22% protein
31% fat

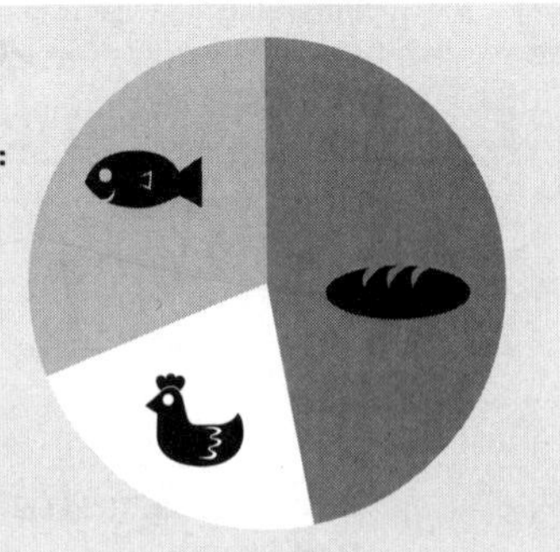

BREAKFAST

- **2 frozen whole grain waffles, toasted, topped with 2 tsp honey and ½ cup raspberries**

Total Calories: 245 kcal
Total Fat: 3.5 g
Saturated Fat: 0 g
Total Carbohydrate: 52 g
Protein: 9 g
Sodium: 331 mg
Fiber: 10 g

NUTRIENT INTAKE:

76% carbs
13% protein
11% fat

SNACK 1

- **1 hard-boiled egg**

Total Calories: 78 kcal
Total Fat: 5 g
Saturated Fat: 1.5 g
Total Carbohydrate: 1 g
Protein: 6 g
Sodium: 62 mg
Fiber: 0 g

NUTRIENT INTAKE:

3% carbs
33% protein
64% fat

LUNCH

- **1½ cups low sodium lentil or black bean soup (Amy's)**
- **2 cups mixed greens topped with 2 Tbsp light vinaigrette salad dressing**

Total Calories: 290 kcal
Total Fat: 10 g
Saturated Fat: 1 g
Total Carbohydrate: 41 g
Protein: 12 g
Sodium: 1001 mg
Fiber: 12 g

NUTRIENT INTAKE:

54% carbs
16% protein
30% fat

SNACK 2

- 1 medium apple
- 1 part-skim mozzarella string cheese

Total Calories: 152 kcal
Total Fat: 6 g
Saturated Fat: 3.5 g
Total Carbohydrate: 20 g
Protein: 7 g
Sodium: 221 mg
Fiber: 3 g

NUTRIENT INTAKE:

48% carbs
18% protein
34% fat

SNACK 3

- ¼ cup cashews

Total Calories: 197 kcal
Total Fat: 16 g
Saturated Fat: 3 g
Total Carbohydrate: 11 g
Protein: 5 g
Sodium: 6 mg
Fiber: 1 g

NUTRIENT INTAKE:

23% carbs
9% protein
68% fat

DINNER

- 5 oz broiled salmon with freshly squeezed lemon juice
- 1 cup steamed zucchini

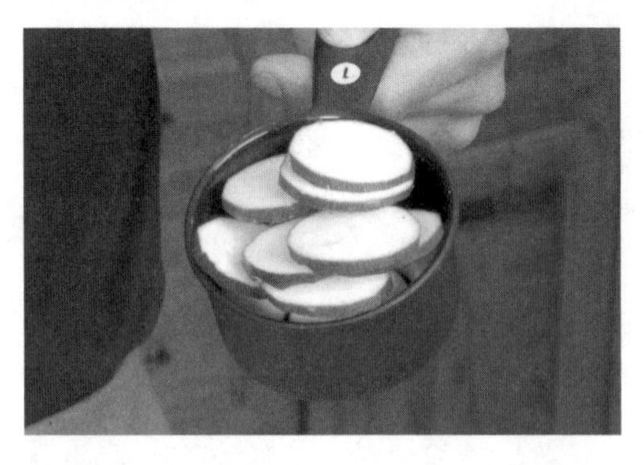

Total Calories: 235 kcal
Total Fat: 6 g
Saturated Fat: 1.5 g
Total Carbohydrate: 9 g
Protein: 35 g
Sodium: 656 mg
Fiber: 3 g

NUTRIENT INTAKE:

16% carbs
60% protein
24% fat

SNACK 4 (OPTIONAL)

▸ **½ frozen banana**

Total Calories: 53 kcal
Total Fat: 0 g
Saturated Fat: 0 g
Total Carbohydrate: 13 g
Protein: 1 g
Sodium: 1 mg
Fiber: 2 g

NUTRIENT INTAKE:

93% carbs
4% protein
3% fat

NUTRITION FOR THE DAY

Total Calories: 1249 kcal
Total Fat: 47 g
Saturated Fat: 11 g
Total Carbohydrate: 147 g
Protein: 75 g
Sodium: 2283 mg
Fiber: 31 g

NUTRIENT INTAKE:

45% carbs
22% protein
33% fat

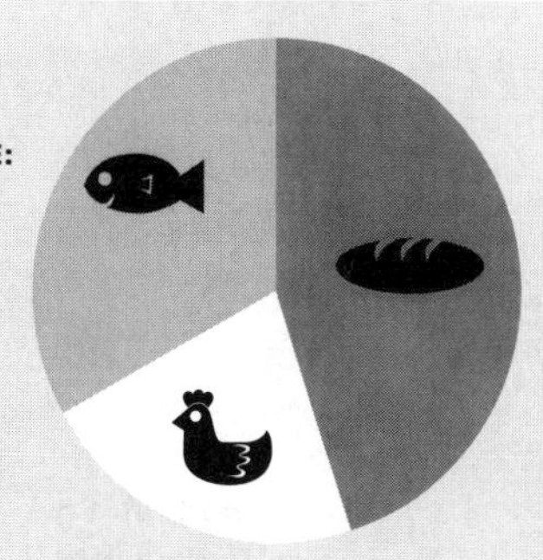

BREAKFAST

- **1 cup whole grain cereal (suggestions: Bran Flakes, Nature's Path Heirloom Flakes)**
- **¾ cup skim milk**
- **½ cup raspberries**

Total Calories: 248 kcal
Total Fat: 2.5 g
Saturated Fat: 0.5 g
Total Carbohydrate: 50 g
Protein: 12 g
Sodium: 79 mg
Fiber: 10 g

NUTRIENT INTAKE:

73% carbs
18% protein
9% fat

SNACK 1

- **10 celery sticks**
- **1 Tbsp almond butter**

Total Calories: 107 kcal
Total Fat: 9.5 g
Saturated Fat: 1 g
Total Carbohydrate: 5 g
Protein: 3 g
Sodium: 104 mg
Fiber: 1 g

NUTRIENT INTAKE:

16% carbs
9% protein
75% fat

LUNCH

- **½ cup cooked whole wheat couscous topped with 2 tsp olive oil and lemon juice and ½ cup chopped tomato, fresh basil, and 3 oz grilled chicken**

Total Calories: 357 kcal
Total Fat: 13 g
Saturated Fat: 2 g
Total Carbohydrate: 31 g
Protein: 32 g
Sodium: 68 mg
Fiber: 4 g

NUTRIENT INTAKE:

34% carbs
35% protein
32% fat

SNACK 2

▸ **1 cup air-popped popcorn**

Total Calories: 31 kcal
Total Fat: 0 g
Saturated Fat: 0 g
Total Carbohydrate: 6 g
Protein: 1 g
Sodium: 1 mg
Fiber: 1 g

NUTRIENT INTAKE:
81% carbs
9% protein
10% fat

SNACK 3

▸ **¼ cup dried apricots**

Total Calories: 100 kcal
Total Fat: 0 g
Saturated Fat: 0 g
Total Carbohydrate: 26 g
Protein: 7 g
Sodium: 62 mg
Fiber: 3 g

NUTRIENT INTAKE:
96% carbs
4% protein
0% fat

DINNER

▸ **Teriyaki chicken salad**

Teriyaki Chicken Salad

SERVES: 1

4 oz boneless, skinless chicken breast
1 Tbsp teriyaki sauce

2 cups mixed greens
½ cup finely diced pineapple
½ cup sliced cucumber
1 Tbsp chopped scallions
1 Tbsp chopped cashews
4 black olives, sliced

Dressing:
2 Tbsp freshly squeezed lime juice
2 tsp canola oil
1 tsp reduced sodium soy sauce
1 tsp honey
½ tsp Dijon mustard
1 Tbsp fresh basil

1. Preheat a grill or grill pan to medium-high.
2. Baste chicken with teriyaki sauce and grill for 4 to 6 minutes per side until cooked through.
3. While the chicken is cooking, place greens in a large bowl and top with pineapple, cucumber, scallions, cashews, and olives.
4. In a small bowl, combine ingredients for dressing and whisk well to combine. Top salad with chicken and dressing and serve.

Total Calories: 414 kcal
Total Fat: 19 g
Saturated Fat: 2 g
Total Carbohydrate: 34 g
Protein: 31 g
Sodium: 888 mg
Fiber: 3 g

NUTRIENT INTAKE:

31% carbs
29% protein
40% fat

SNACK 4 (OPTIONAL)

- **1 small container sugar-free gelatin**

Total Calories: 10 kcal
Total Fat: 0 g
Saturated Fat: 0 g
Total Carbohydrate: 0 g
Protein: 1 g
Sodium: 45 mg
Fiber: 0 g

NUTRIENT INTAKE:

0% carbs
100% protein
0% fat

NUTRITION FOR THE DAY

Total Calories: 1267 kcal
Total Fat: 44 g
Saturated Fat: 5.5 g
Total Carbohydrate: 151 g
Protein: 81 g
Sodium: 1185 mg
Fiber: 23 g

NUTRIENT INTAKE:

47% carbs
29% protein
24% fat

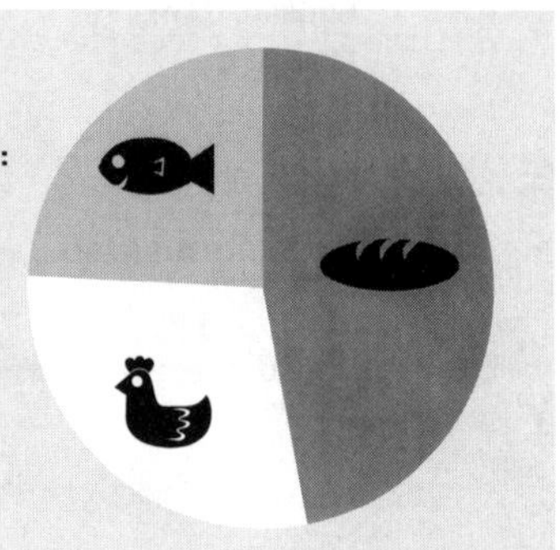

BREAKFAST

- **1 slice whole wheat bread, toasted**
- **1 Tbsp almond butter**

Total Calories: 211 kcal
Total Fat: 11 g
Saturated Fat: 1.5 g
Total Carbohydrate: 23 g
Protein: 6 g
Sodium: 222 mg
Fiber: 4 g

NUTRIENT INTAKE:

43% carbs
12% protein
45% fat

SNACK 1

- **½ cup sliced mango**

Total Calories: 54 kcal
Total Fat: 0 g
Saturated Fat: 0 g
Total Carbohydrate: 14 g
Protein: 0 g
Sodium: 2 mg
Fiber: 1 g

NUTRIENT INTAKE:

94% carbs
3% protein
3% fat

LUNCH

- **Garden Salad with Egg**

2 cups mixed greens
½ cup sliced cucumber
¼ cup chopped tomato
1 hard-boiled egg
¼ cup canned chickpeas, rinsed and drained
2 tsp olive oil and 1 Tbsp balsamic vinegar

Total Calories: 261 kcal
Total Fat: 15 g
Saturated Fat: 3 g
Total Carbohydrate: 22 g
Protein: 11 g
Sodium: 270 mg
Fiber: 4 g

NUTRIENT INTAKE:

32% carbs
17% protein
51% fat

SNACK 2

- 1 medium apple

Total Calories: 72 kcal
Total Fat: 0 g
Saturated Fat: 0 g
Total Carbohydrate: 19 g
Protein: 0 g
Sodium: 1 mg
Fiber: 3 g

NUTRIENT INTAKE:

96% carbs
2% protein
2% fat

SNACK 3

- 2 oz low sodium roast beef

Total Calories: 90 kcal
Total Fat: 3 g
Saturated Fat: 1.5 g
Total Carbohydrate: 0 g
Protein: 14 g
Sodium: 40 mg
Fiber: 0 g

NUTRIENT INTAKE:

0% carbs
67% protein
33% fat

DINNER

- 4 oz grilled shrimp (make a double batch for lunch on Day 7)
- 1 cup cooked whole wheat pasta with 1 cup steamed Swiss chard and 2 tsp olive oil

Total Calories: 400 kcal
Total Fat: 11 g
Saturated Fat: 2 g
Total Carbohydrate: 44 g
Protein: 34 g
Sodium: 572 mg
Fiber: 10 g

NUTRIENT INTAKE:

81% carbs
15% protein
4% fat

SNACK 4 (OPTIONAL)

- **½ frozen banana**

Total Calories: 53 kcal
Total Fat: 0 g
Saturated Fat: 0 g
Total Carbohydrate: 13 g
Protein: 1 g
Sodium: 1 mg
Fiber: 2 g

NUTRIENT INTAKE:

93% carbs
4% protein
3% fat

NUTRITION FOR THE DAY

Total Calories: 1141 kcal
Total Fat: 41 g
Saturated Fat: 8 g
Total Carbohydrate: 136 g
Protein: 67 g
Sodium: 1107 mg
Fiber: 25 g

NUTRIENT INTAKE:

63% carbs
17% protein
20% fat

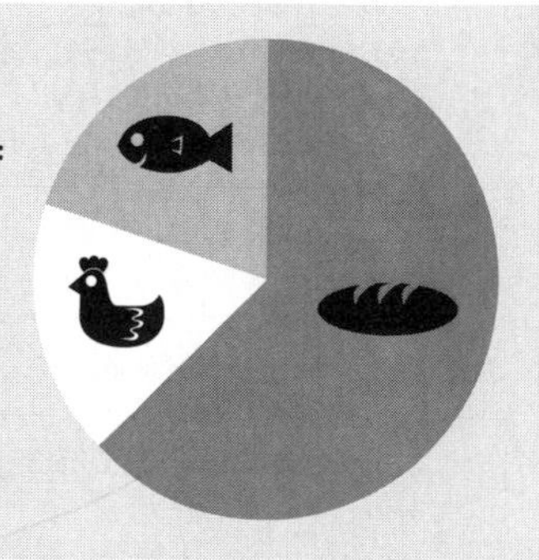

BREAKFAST

- **1 slice whole wheat bread, toasted**
- **Tomato and Swiss omelet**

Tomato and Swiss Omelet

SERVES: 1

Nonstick cooking spray
1 egg
2 egg whites
1 Tbsp water
¼ cup arugula, finely chopped
¼ cup chopped tomato
1 slice low fat Swiss cheese
Salt and pepper to taste

1. Heat a nonstick skillet over medium heat.
2. Combine egg, egg whites, and water in a bowl, season with salt and pepper and whisk well.
3. Add tomato and arugula to eggs.
4. Spray skillet with nonstick spray and add egg mixture.
5. Cook for 3 to 4 minutes until eggs begin to set. Using a rubber spatula, gently pull in the sides of the omelet to let the uncooked egg run to the edges of the pan.
6. Place cheese on one side of the omelet and gently fold in half. Allow to cook for 2 minutes until cheese is melted. Slide omelet onto a plate.

Total Calories: 277 kcal
Total Fat: 8 g
Saturated Fat: 3 g
Total Carbohydrate: 24 g
Protein: 26 g
Sodium: 406 mg
Fiber: 4 g

NUTRIENT INTAKE:

35% carbs
38% protein
27% fat

SNACK 1

- **1 medium banana**

Total Calories: 105 kcal
Total Fat: 0 g
Saturated Fat: 0 g
Total Carbohydrate: 27 g
Protein: 1 g
Sodium: 1 mg
Fiber: 3 g

NUTRIENT INTAKE:

93% carbs
4% protein
3% fat

LUNCH

▸ Roast Beef and Swiss Wrap

1 whole wheat tortilla (6 inch)
3 oz low sodium roast beef
1 slice low fat Swiss cheese
2 slices tomato
2 tsp Dijon mustard
½ cup fresh arugula

Total Calories: 338 kcal
Total Fat: 9 g
Saturated Fat: 3 g
Total Carbohydrate: 25 g
Protein: 33 g
Sodium: 546 mg
Fiber: 3 g

NUTRIENT INTAKE:

32% carbs
42% protein
26% fat

SNACK 2

▸ ½ cup raspberries

Total Calories: 40 kcal
Total Fat: 0 g
Saturated Fat: 0 g
Total Carbohydrate: 9 g
Protein: 1 g
Sodium: 1 mg
Fiber: 5 g

NUTRIENT INTAKE:

82% carbs
8% protein
10% fat

SNACK 3

▸ 1 part-skim mozzarella string cheese

Total Calories: 80 kcal
Total Fat: 6 g
Saturated Fat: 3.5 g
Total Carbohydrate: 1 g
Protein: 7 g
Sodium: 220 mg
Fiber: 0 g

NUTRIENT INTAKE:

5% carbs
33% protein
62% fat

DINNER

- 3 oz grilled turkey breast
- ¾ cup cooked whole wheat couscous
- 1 cup sliced cucumber topped with 1 Tbsp light vinaigrette salad dressing

Turkey breast cutlets are just as lean and as high in protein as chicken breasts.

Total Calories: 293 kcal
Total Fat: 3 g
Saturated Fat: 0 g
Total Carbohydrate: 40 g
Protein: 28 g
Sodium: 278 mg
Fiber: 4 g

NUTRIENT INTAKE:

53% carbs
37% protein
10% fat

DESSERT

- 1 oz dark chocolate

The darker the chocolate, the better for less fat and more antioxidants.

Total Calories: 146 kcal
Total Fat: 9 g
Saturated Fat: 5 g
Total Carbohydrate: 17 g
Protein: 2 g
Sodium: 0 mg
Fiber: 2 g

NUTRIENT INTAKE:

43% carbs
4% protein
53% fat

NUTRITION FOR THE DAY

Total Calories: 1271 kcal
Total Fat: 36 g
Saturated Fat: 15 g
Total Carbohydrate: 141 g
Protein: 97 g
Sodium: 1452 mg
Fiber: 20 g

NUTRIENT INTAKE:

49% carbs

24% protein

27% fat

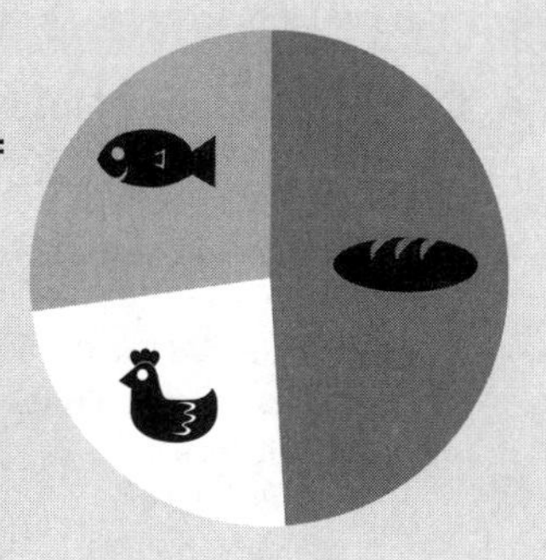

BREAKFAST

- **1 cup cooked oatmeal topped with 2 Tbsp chopped dried apricots and 1 Tbsp toasted wheat germ**

Total Calories: 222 kcal
Total Fat: 3 g
Saturated Fat: 0 g
Total Carbohydrate: 41 g
Protein: 9 g
Sodium: 2 mg
Fiber: 6 g

NUTRIENT INTAKE:
73% carbs
15% protein
12% fat

SNACK 1

- **½ cup dry whole grain cereal**
- **1 medium apple**

Total Calories: 148 kcal
Total Fat: 1 g
Saturated Fat: 0 g
Total Carbohydrate: 36 g
Protein: 3 g
Sodium: 2 mg
Fiber: 6 g

NUTRIENT INTAKE:
86% carbs
7% protein
7% fat

LUNCH

- **Grilled Shrimp Caesar Salad**

2 cups romaine lettuce
½ cup sliced cucumber
¼ cup sliced red onion
4 oz grilled shrimp
2 Tbsp light Caesar dressing

Total Calories: 223 kcal
Total Fat: 7.5 g
Saturated Fat: 1 g
Total Carbohydrate: 12 g
Protein: 27 g
Sodium: 784 mg
Fiber: 3 g

NUTRIENT INTAKE:
22% carbs
47% protein
31% fat

SNACK 2

- ½ cup sliced mango

Total Calories: 54 kcal
Total Fat: 0 g
Saturated Fat: 0 g
Total Carbohydrate: 14 g
Protein: 0 g
Sodium: 2 mg
Fiber: 1 g

NUTRIENT INTAKE:

94% carbs
3% protein
3% fat

SNACK 3

- ¼ cup dry roasted cashews

Total Calories: 197 kcal
Total Fat: 16 g
Saturated Fat: 3 g
Total Carbohydrate: 11 g
Protein: 5 g
Sodium: 6 mg
Fiber: 1 g

NUTRIENT INTAKE:

23% carbs
9% protein
68% fat

DINNER

- 1 cup butternut squash roasted with 1 tsp olive oil, salt and pepper
- 1½ cups mixed greens topped with 1 tsp olive oil and lemon juice
- Baked chicken cutlets

QUICK OPTION MEAL for baked chicken cutlets < < < < < < <

4 oz grilled chicken breast

Total Calories: 187 kcal
Total Fat: 4 g
Saturated Fat: 1.5 g
Total Carbohydrate: 0 g
Protein: 35 g
Sodium: 84 mg
Fiber: 0 g

NUTRITION INTAKE:

0% carbs
81% protein
19% fat

Baked Chicken Cutlets

SERVES: 4

4 thinly sliced chicken breast cutlets (3 oz each)
½ cup flour
1 egg, lightly beaten
½ cup seasoned bread crumbs
¼ cup grated Parmesan cheese
½ cup panko bread crumbs
1 Tbsp canola oil
Salt and pepper
Cooking spray

1. Preheat oven to 400°F.
2. Set up a breading station with 3 shallow bowls. Place flour in one bowl; whisk egg in a separate bowl; and in the final bowl, combine bread crumbs and Parmesan cheese.
3. Season all three bowls with salt and pepper.
4. Toss chicken in flour, shake off excess and transfer to egg, and then to bread crumb mixture.
5. Brush a baking sheet with canola oil.
6. Place chicken on oiled baking sheet and spray with nonstick spray. Place in oven and cook for 15 to 20 minutes, turning once until golden and crisp.

Baking instead of frying will save more than 150 calories per serving.

Total Calories: 388 kcal
Total Fat: 16 g
Saturated Fat: 2.5 g
Total Carbohydrate: 37 g
Protein: 27 g
Sodium: 804 mg
Fiber: 1 g

NUTRIENT INTAKE:

37% carbs
27% protein
36% fat

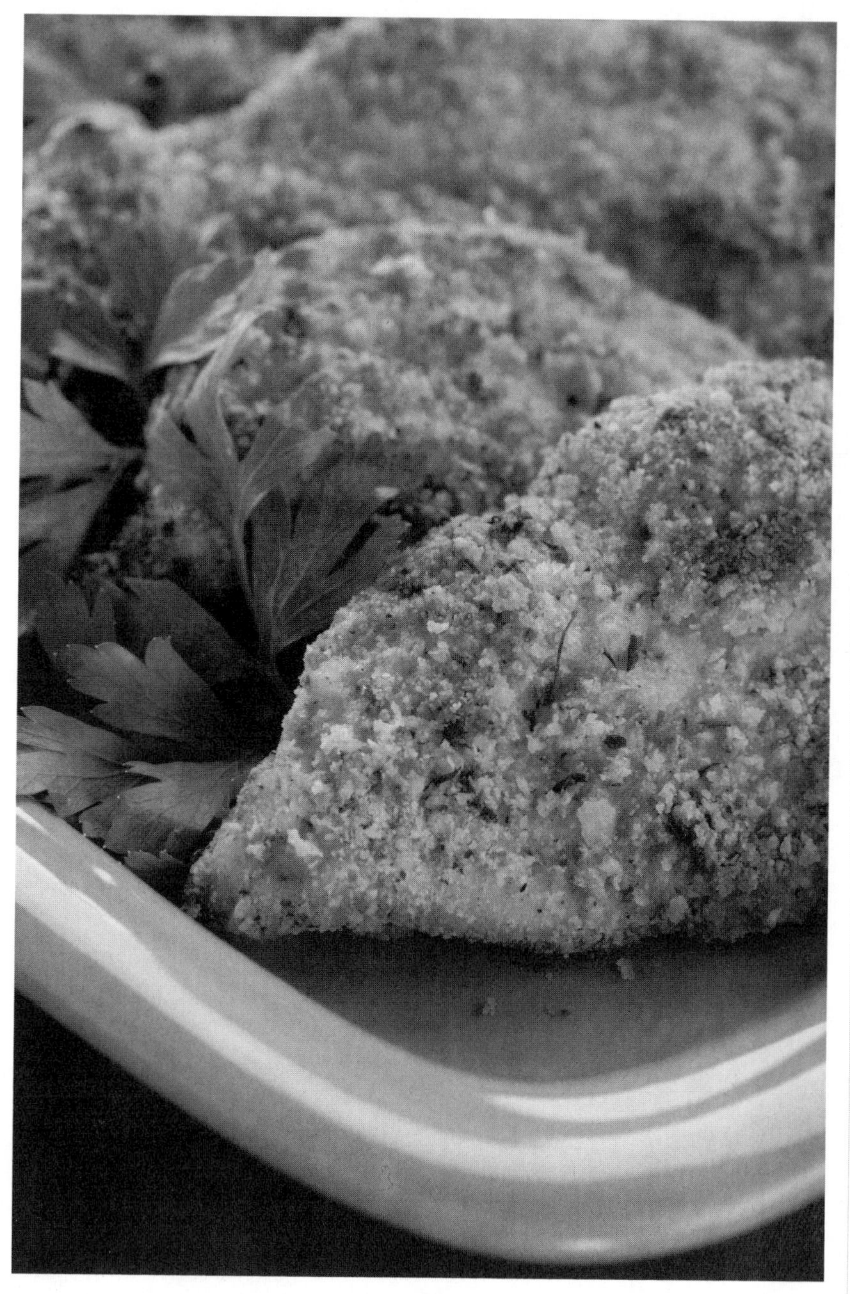

SNACK 4 (OPTIONAL)

- ½ cup frozen pineapple

Total Calories: 37 kcal
Total Fat: 0 g
Saturated Fat: 0 g
Total Carbohydrate: 10 g
Protein: 0 g
Sodium: 1 mg
Fiber: 1 g

NUTRIENT INTAKE:

94% carbs
4% protein
2% fat

NUTRITION FOR THE DAY

Total Calories: 1270 kcal
Total Fat: 44 g
Saturated Fat: 8 g
Total Carbohydrate: 161 g
Protein: 71 g
Sodium: 1600 mg
Fiber: 21 g

NUTRIENT INTAKE:

61% carbs
16% protein
23% fat

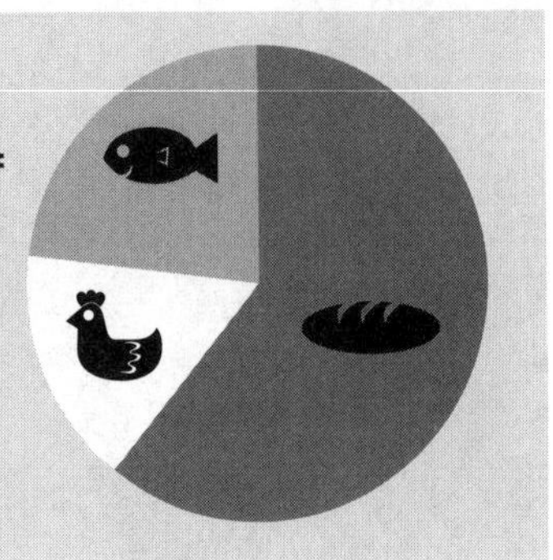

BREAKFAST

- 1 cup nonfat Greek yogurt topped with ½ cup blueberries, 1 tsp lemon zest, and 1 Tbsp toasted wheat germ
- 1 hard-boiled egg

There's just as much protein in an egg yolk as in an egg white.

Total Calories: 266 kcal
Total Fat: 6 g
Saturated Fat: 2 g
Total Carbohydrate: 24 g
Protein: 29 g
Sodium: 148 mg
Fiber: 3 g

NUTRIENT INTAKE:

35% carbs
44% protein
21% fat

SNACK 1

- 1 medium pear
- 1 oz low fat cheddar cheese

Total Calories: 145 kcal
Total Fat: 2 g
Saturated Fat: 1 g
Total Carbohydrate: 26 g
Protein: 8 g
Sodium: 175 mg
Fiber: 5 g

NUTRIENT INTAKE:

68% carbs
19% protein
13% fat

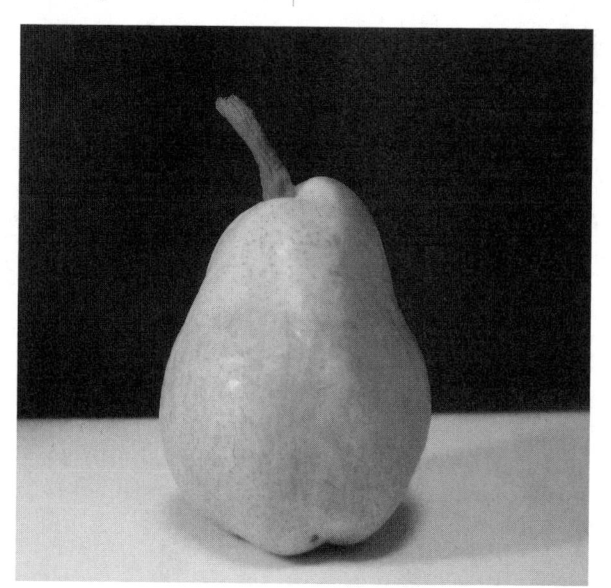

LUNCH

▸ **Bulgur salad**

Bulgur Salad

SERVES: 2

¼ cup bulgur wheat
⅓ cup boiling water
Pinch salt
1 tsp olive oil
1 tsp lemon juice

1 cup diced cooked chicken
½ cup diced cucumber
¼ cup canned chickpeas, rinsed and drained
¼ cup frozen corn, thawed
5 olives, chopped
1 Tbsp chopped fresh parsley

1. Combine bulgur, boiling water, salt, olive oil, and lemon juice in a bowl.
2. Cover with plastic wrap and set aside for 20 to 30 minutes until water is absorbed and bulgur is tender.
3. Add remaining ingredients and mix well to combine.

Bulgur wheat is a chewy and nutty grain with protein, fiber, and iron.

Total Calories: 267 kcal
Total Fat: 6.5 g
Saturated Fat: 1 g
Total Carbohydrate: 26 g
Protein: 26 g
Sodium: 345 mg
Fiber: 5 g

NUTRIENT INTAKE:

38% carbs
39% protein
23% fat

SNACK 2

- **1 medium orange**

Total Calories: 62 kcal
Total Fat: 0 g
Saturated Fat: 0 g
Total Carbohydrate: 15 g
Protein: 6 g
Sodium: 0 mg
Fiber: 6 g

NUTRIENT INTAKE:

90% carbs
7% protein
3% fat

SNACK 3

- **20 almonds**

Packed with protein, fiber, and healthy fat, almonds make for a healthy and satisfying snack.

Total Calories: 139 kcal
Total Fat: 12 g
Saturated Fat: 1 g
Total Carbohydrate: 5 g
Protein: 5 g
Sodium: 0 mg
Fiber: 6 g

NUTRIENT INTAKE:

14% carbs
13% protein
73% fat

DINNER

- **4 oz grilled chicken sausage (1 or 2 links depending on brand)—(freeze remaining for next week)**
- **2 cups steamed broccoli with lemon**

Total Calories: 278 kcal
Total Fat: 11 g
Saturated Fat: 3.5 g
Total Carbohydrate: 26 g
Protein: 26 g
Sodium: 787 mg
Fiber: 10 g

NUTRIENT INTAKE:

33% carbs
34% protein
33% fat

SNACK 4 (OPTIONAL)

- **2 brown rice cakes (any flavor)**

Brown rice cakes have more fiber and protein than the regular kind.

Total Calories: 70 kcal
Total Fat: 0.5 g
Saturated Fat: 0 g
Total Carbohydrate: 15 g
Protein: 1 g
Sodium: 59 mg
Fiber: 1 g

NUTRIENT INTAKE:

87% carbs
7% protein
6% fat

NUTRITION FOR THE DAY

Total Calories: 1226 kcal
Total Fat: 39.5 g
Saturated Fat: 9 g
Total Carbohydrate: 136 g
Protein: 96 g
Sodium: 1514 mg
Fiber: 30 g

NUTRIENT INTAKE:

52% carbs
23% protein
25% fat

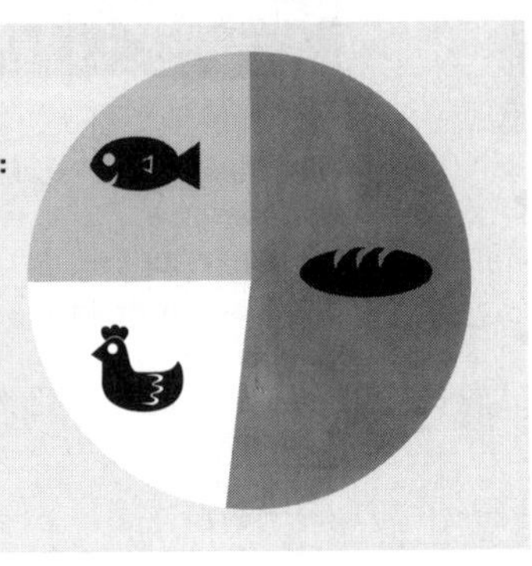

BREAKFAST

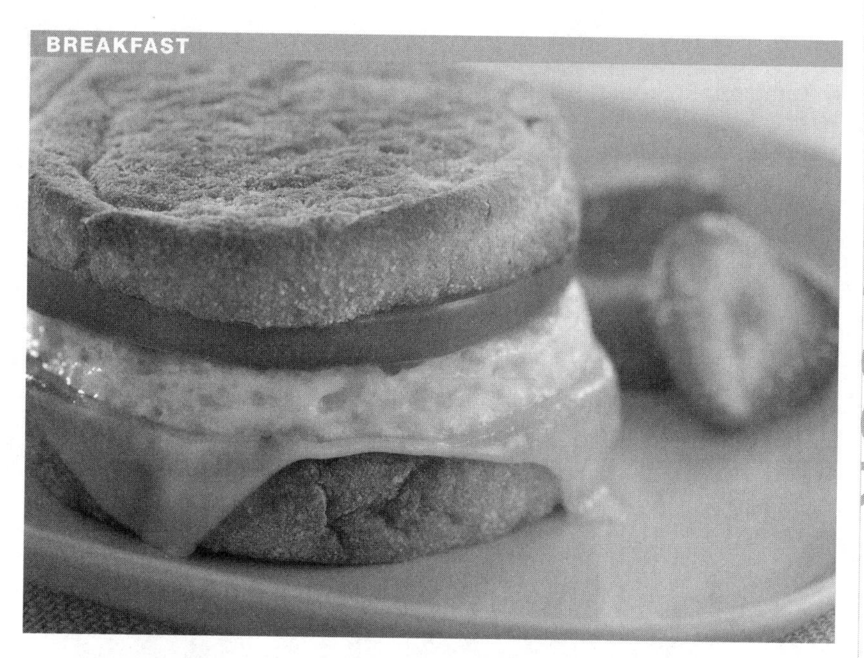

- **Egg Sandwich**
  Whole wheat English muffin
  1 egg, scrambled with ½ cup chopped baby spinach
- **1 medium orange**

Total Calories: 276 kcal
Total Fat: 6.5 g
Saturated Fat: 2 g
Total Carbohydrate: 43 g
Protein: 14 g
Sodium: 512 mg
Fiber: 8 g

NUTRIENT INTAKE:

60% carbs
20% protein
20% fat

SNACK 1

- **10 cherry tomatoes**
- **2 Tbsp hummus**

Total Calories: 77 kcal
Total Fat: 3 g
Saturated Fat: 0.5 g
Total Carbohydrate: 11 g
Protein: 4 g
Sodium: 115 mg
Fiber: 4 g

NUTRIENT INTAKE:

50% carbs
18% protein
32% fat

LUNCH

▸ Guacamole Salad with Chicken

2 cups chopped lettuce
½ cup chopped bell pepper
5 cherry tomatoes, halved
2 Tbsp diced avocado
1 Tbsp fresh cilantro (optional)
4 oz grilled chicken breast, sliced
1 tsp olive oil
Fresh lime juice to taste

Avocado is a great source of heart-healthy monounsaturated fats.

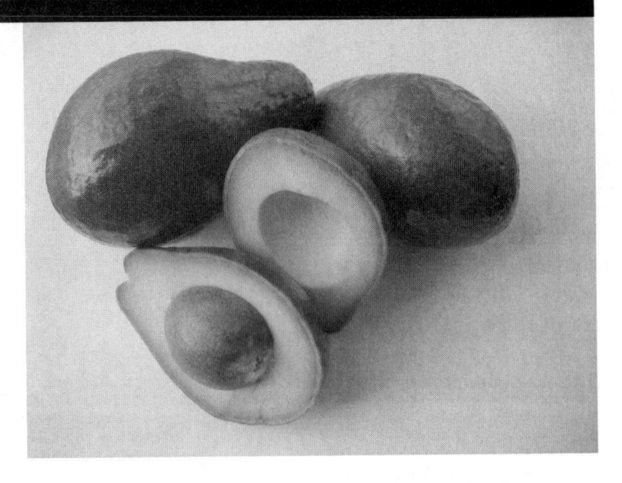

Total Calories: 308 kcal
Total Fat: 12 g
Saturated Fat: 2 g
Total Carbohydrate: 13 g
Protein: 39 g
Sodium: 97 mg
Fiber: 5 g

NUTRIENT INTAKE:

16% carbs
50% protein
34% fat

SNACK 2

▸ 1 medium orange

Total Calories: 62 kcal
Total Fat: 0 g
Saturated Fat: 0 g
Total Carbohydrate: 15 g
Protein: 1 g
Sodium: 0 mg
Fiber: 3 g

NUTRIENT INTAKE:

90% carbs
7% protein
3% fat

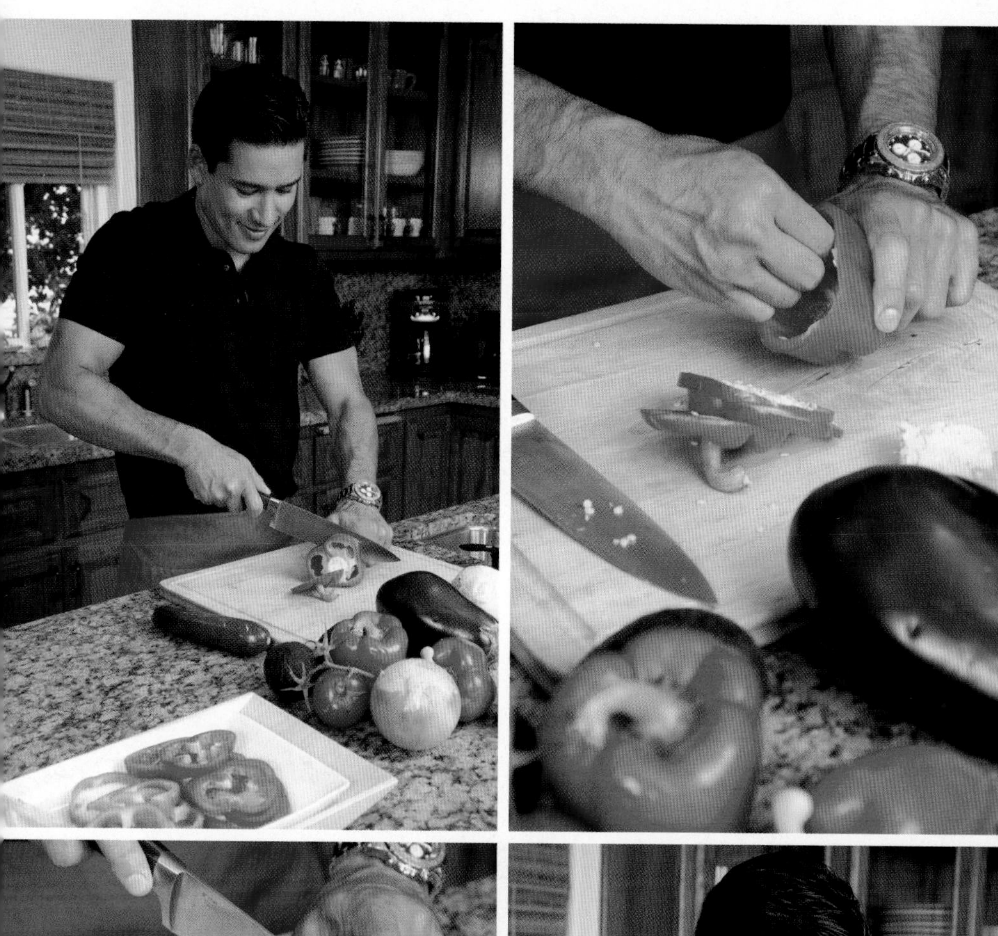

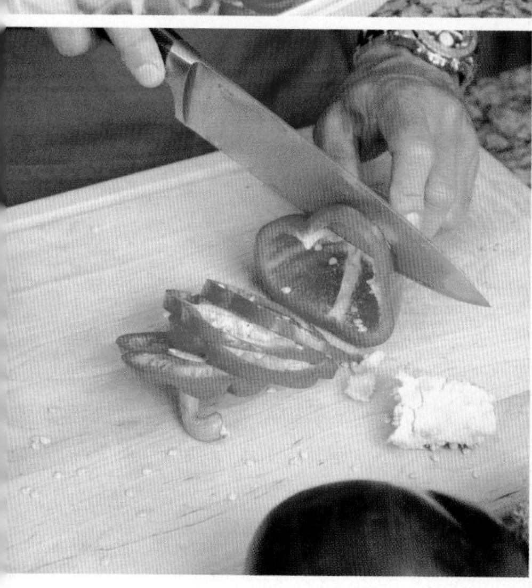

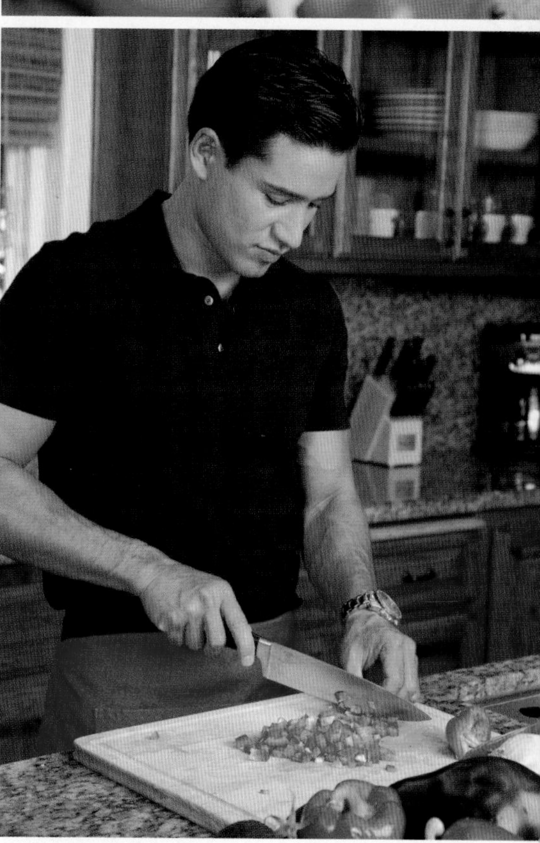

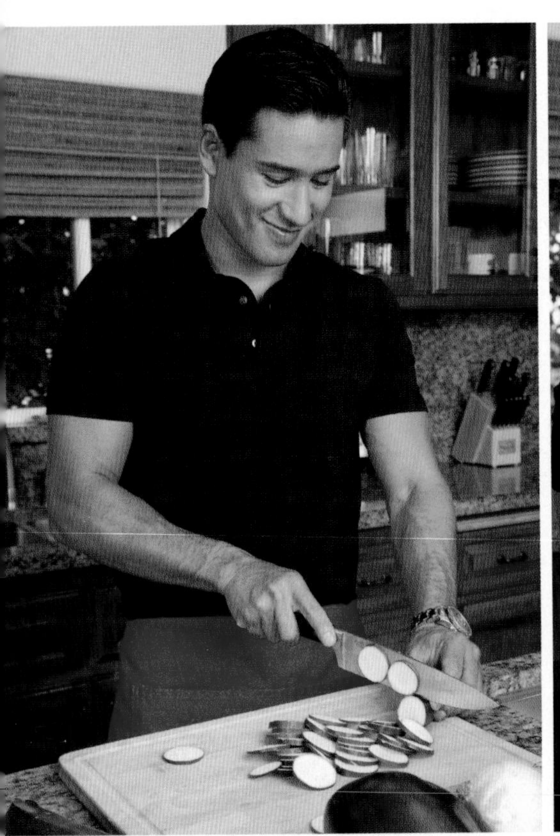

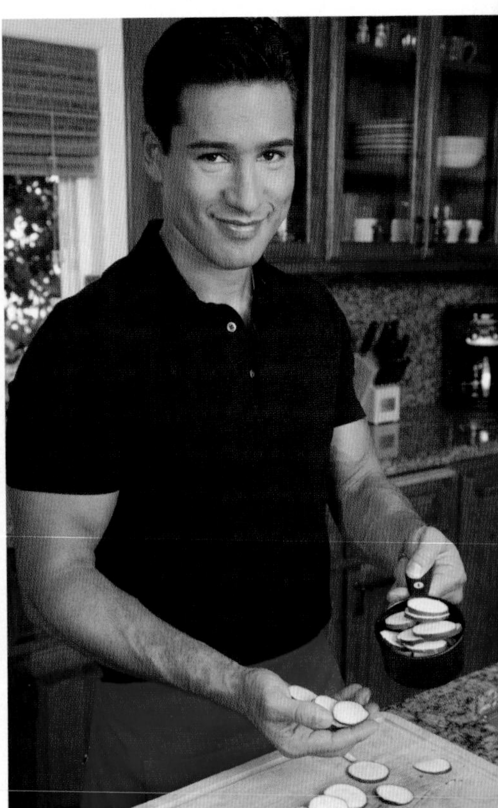

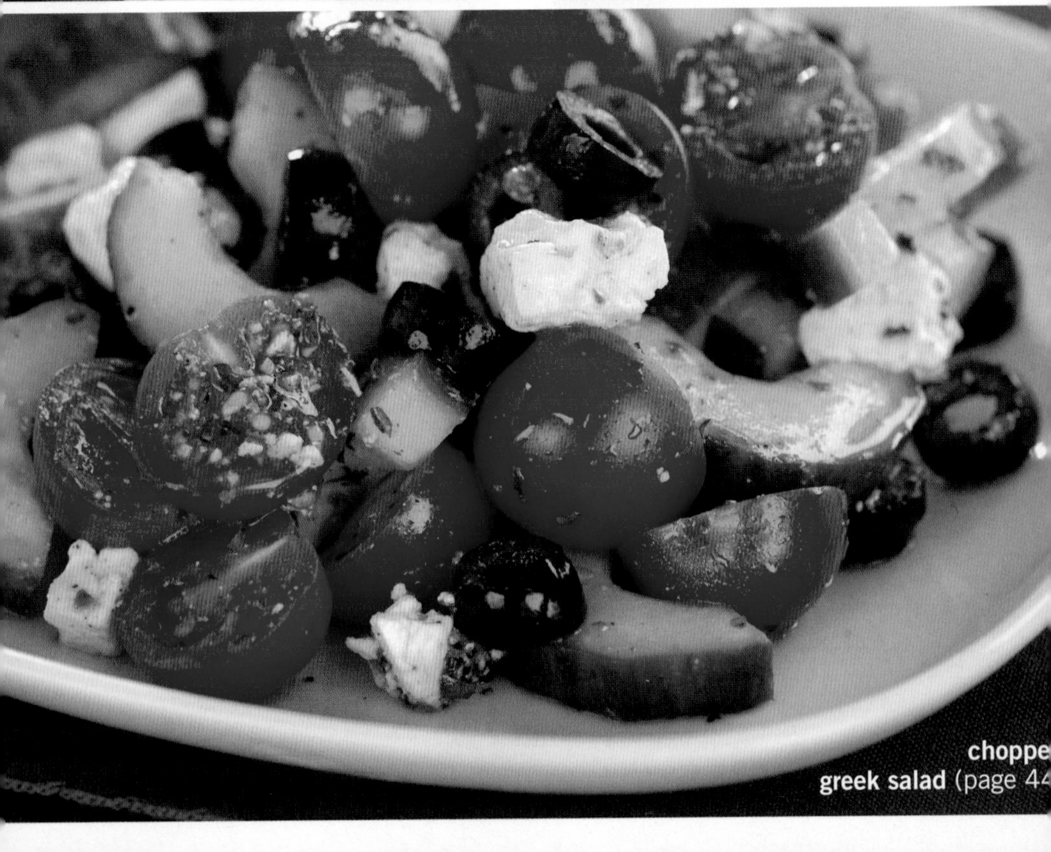

choppe
greek salad (page 44

guacamole salad with chicken (page 118)

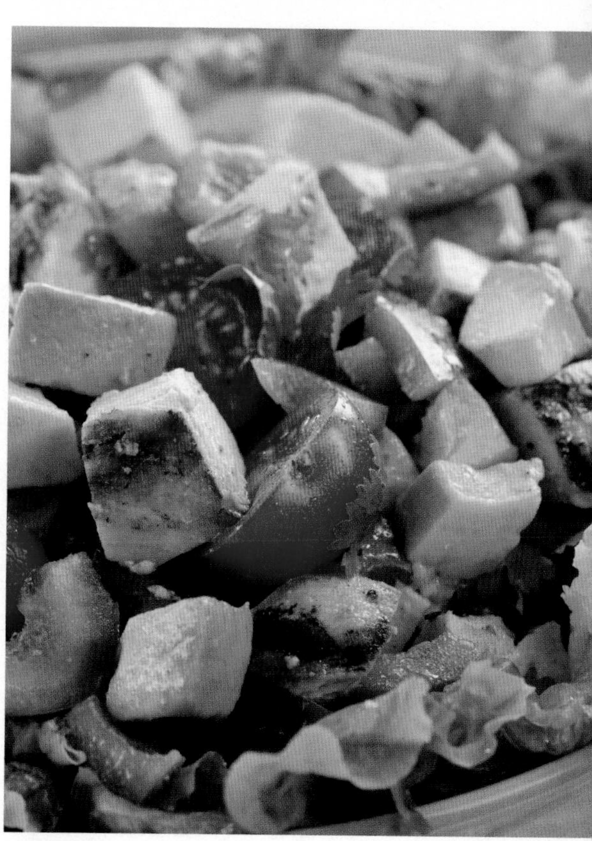

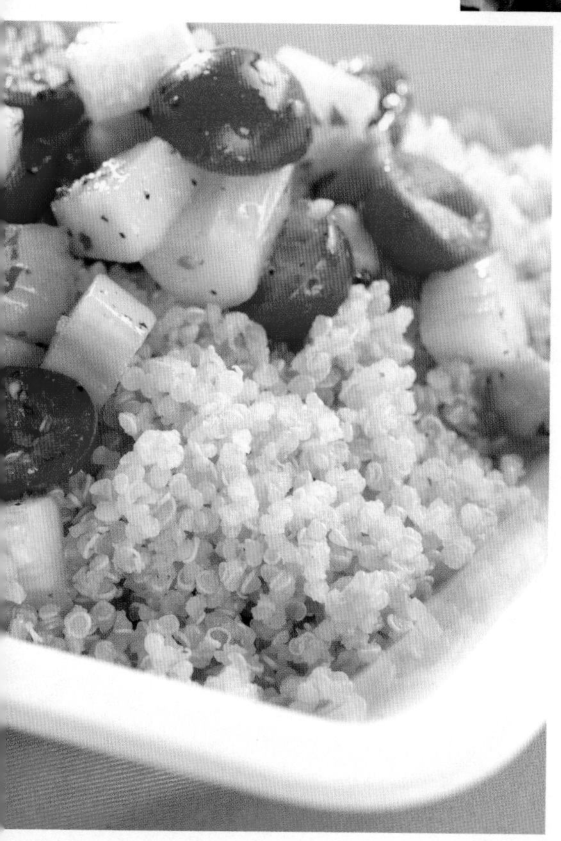

quinoa salad (page 71)

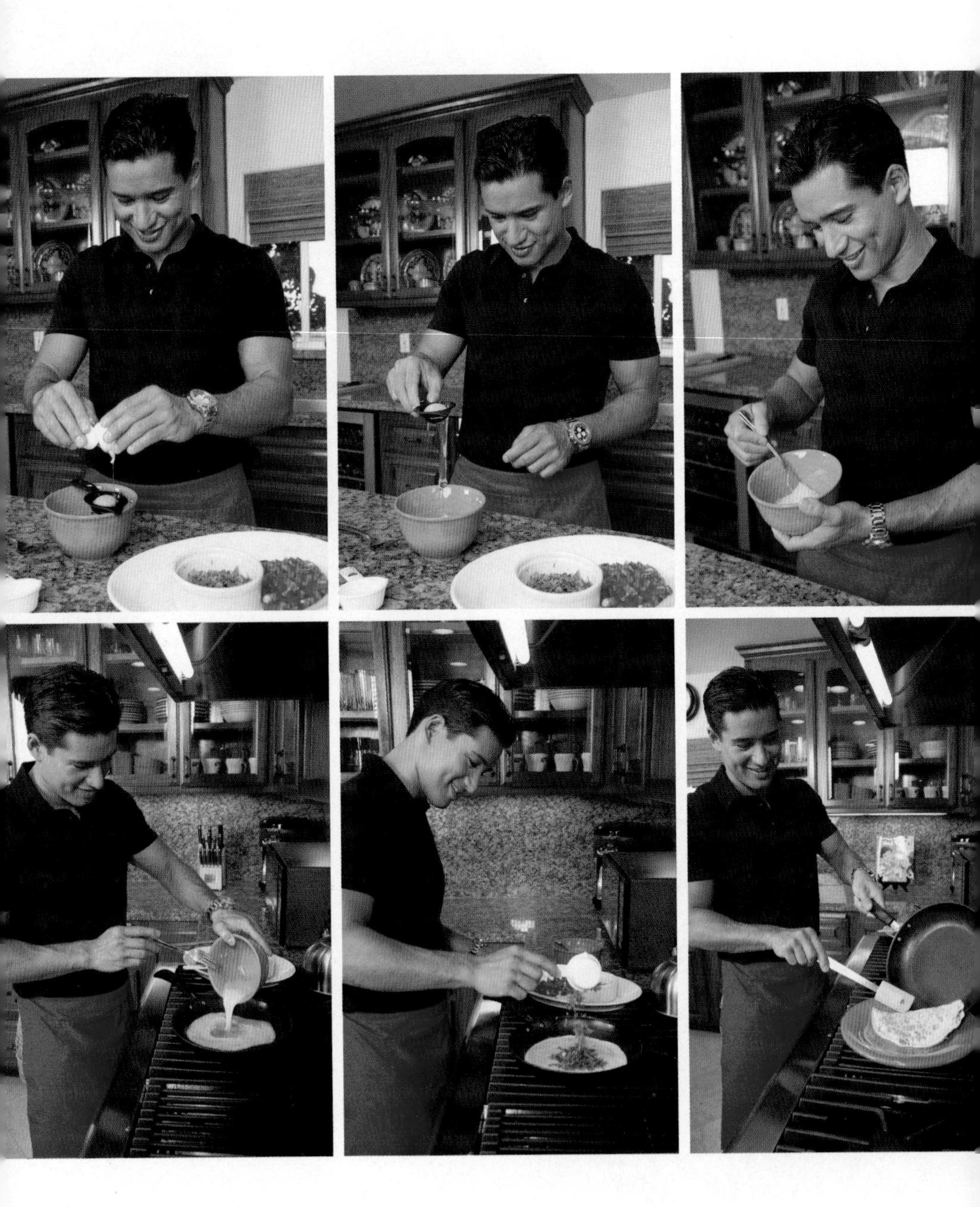

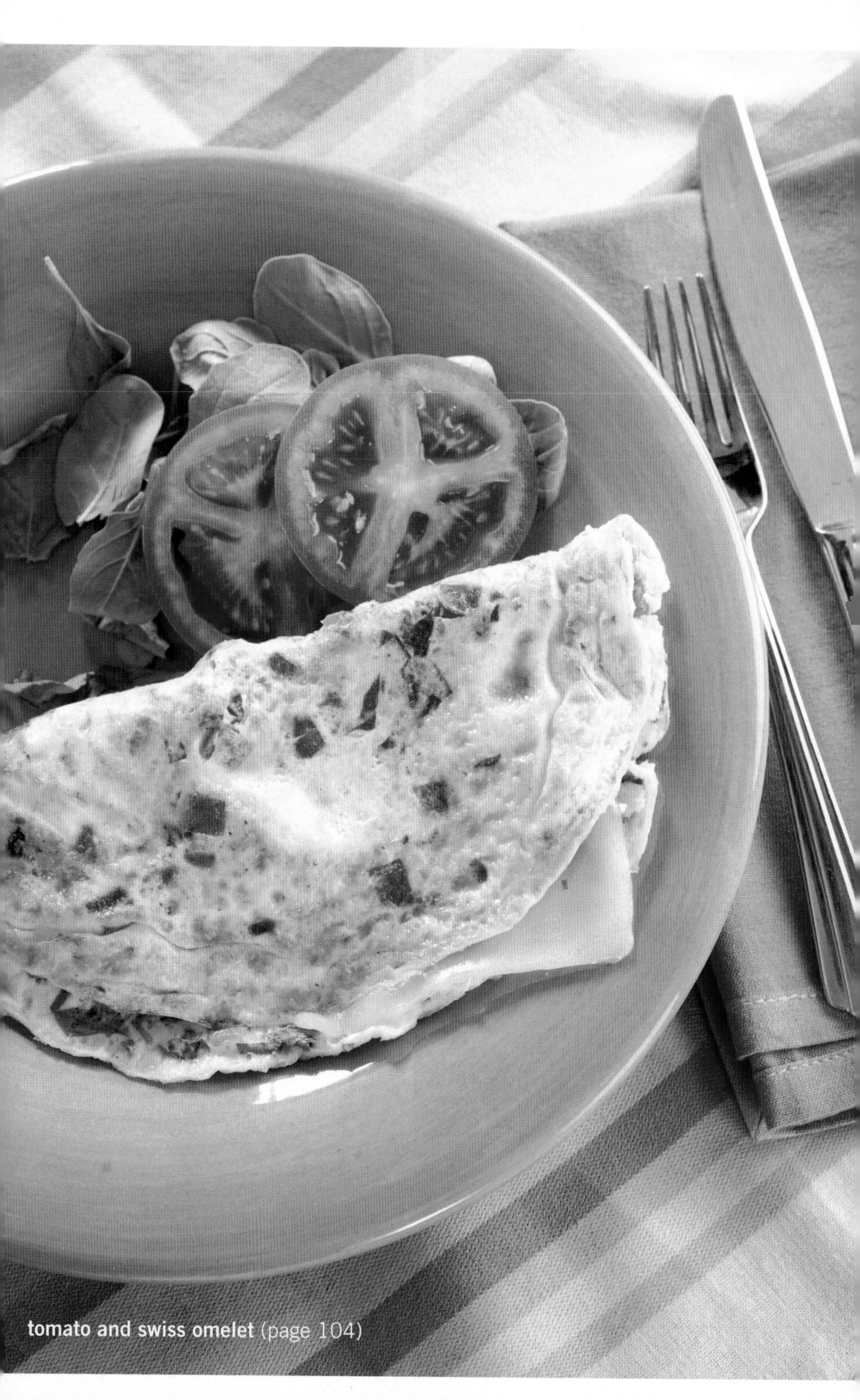

tomato and swiss omelet (page 104)

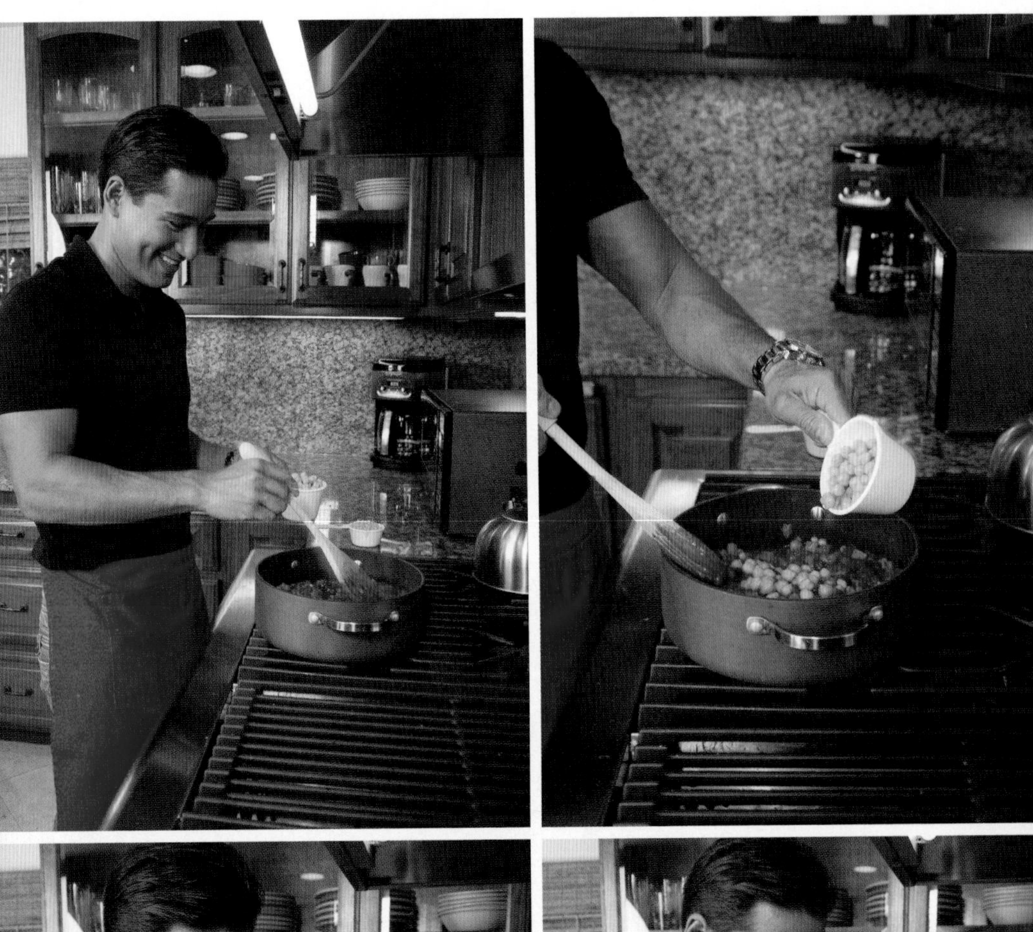
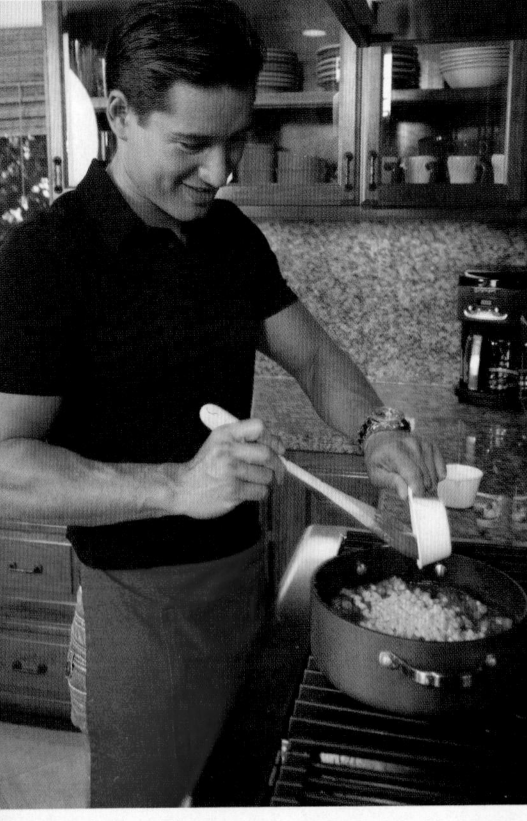
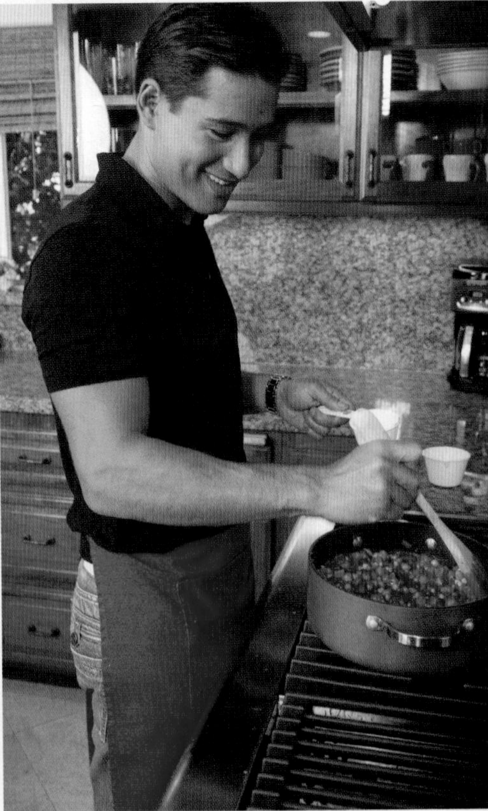

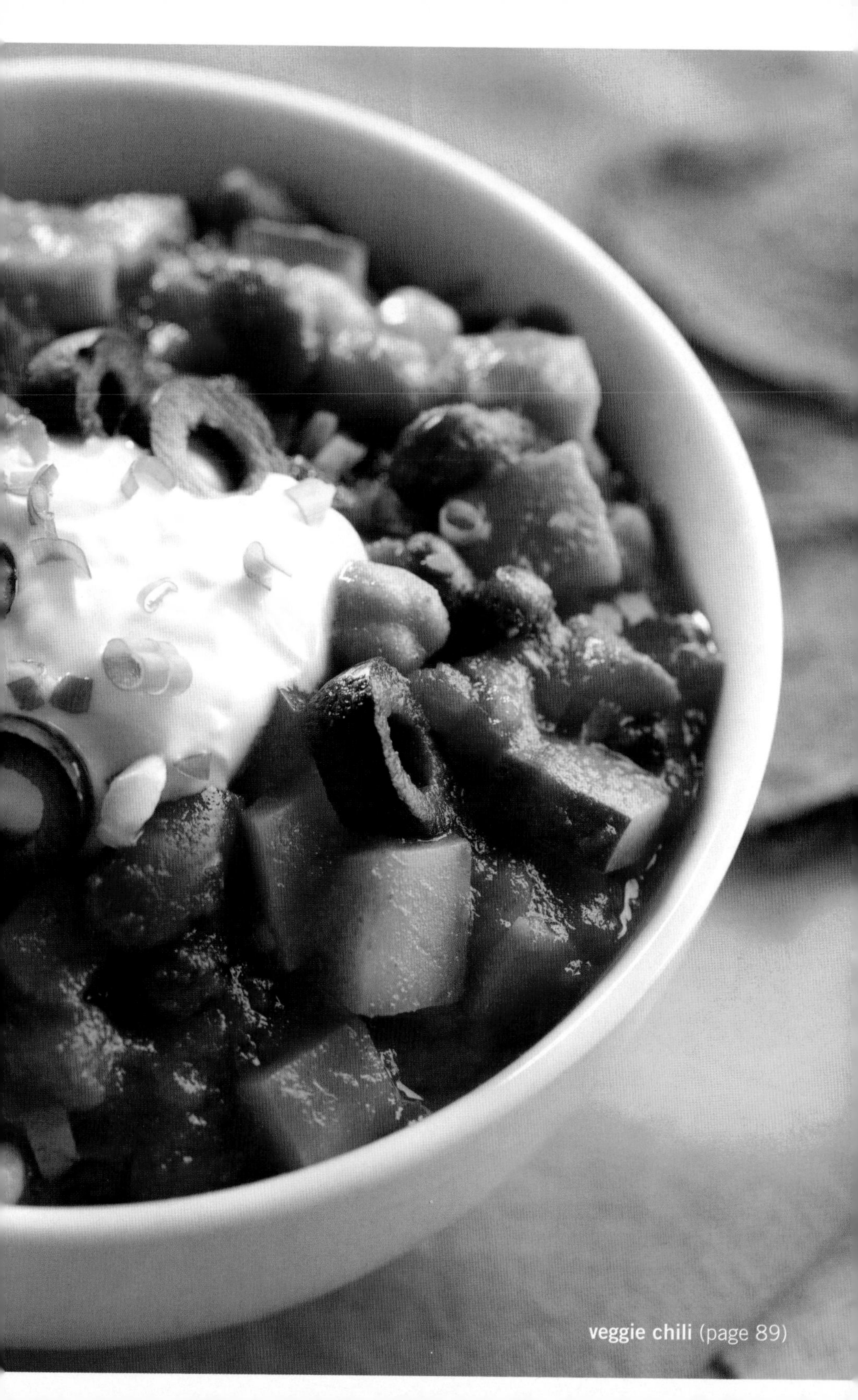

veggie chili (page 89)

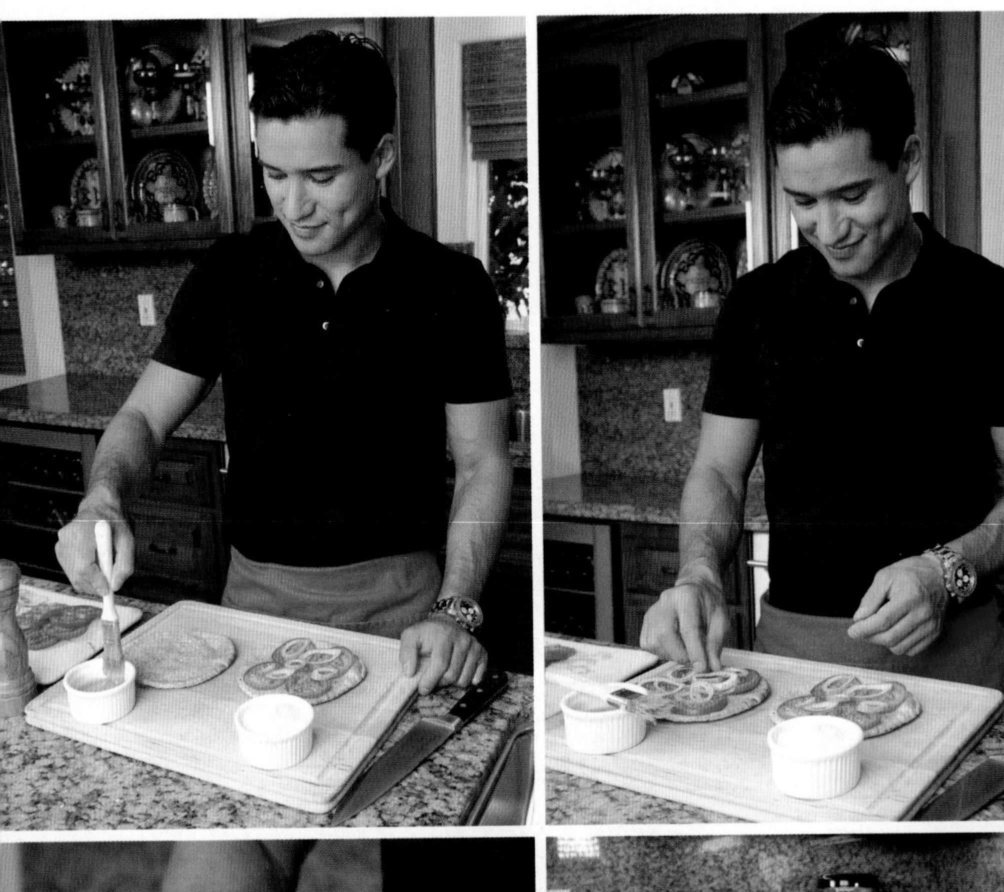
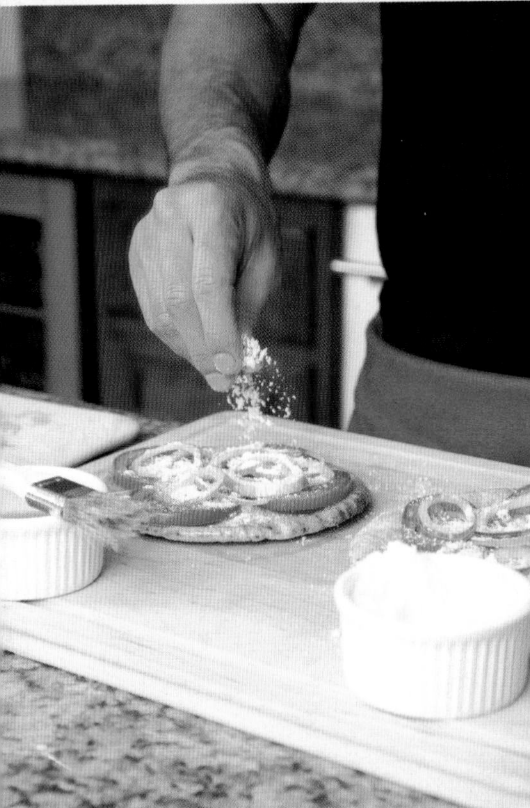
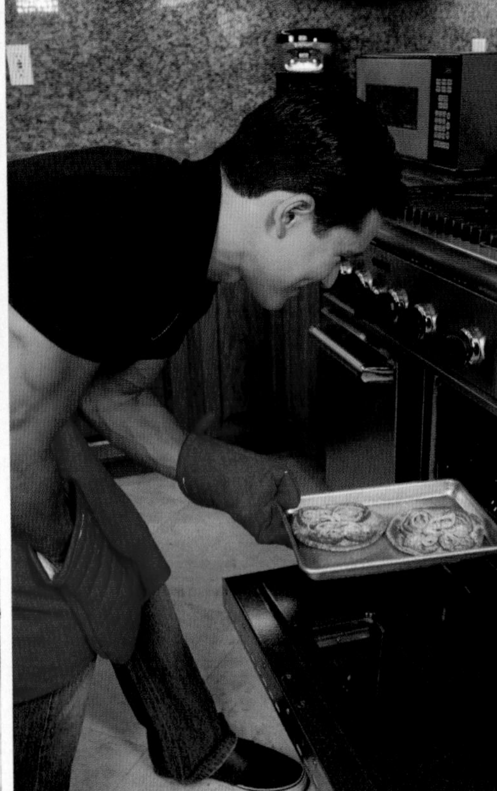

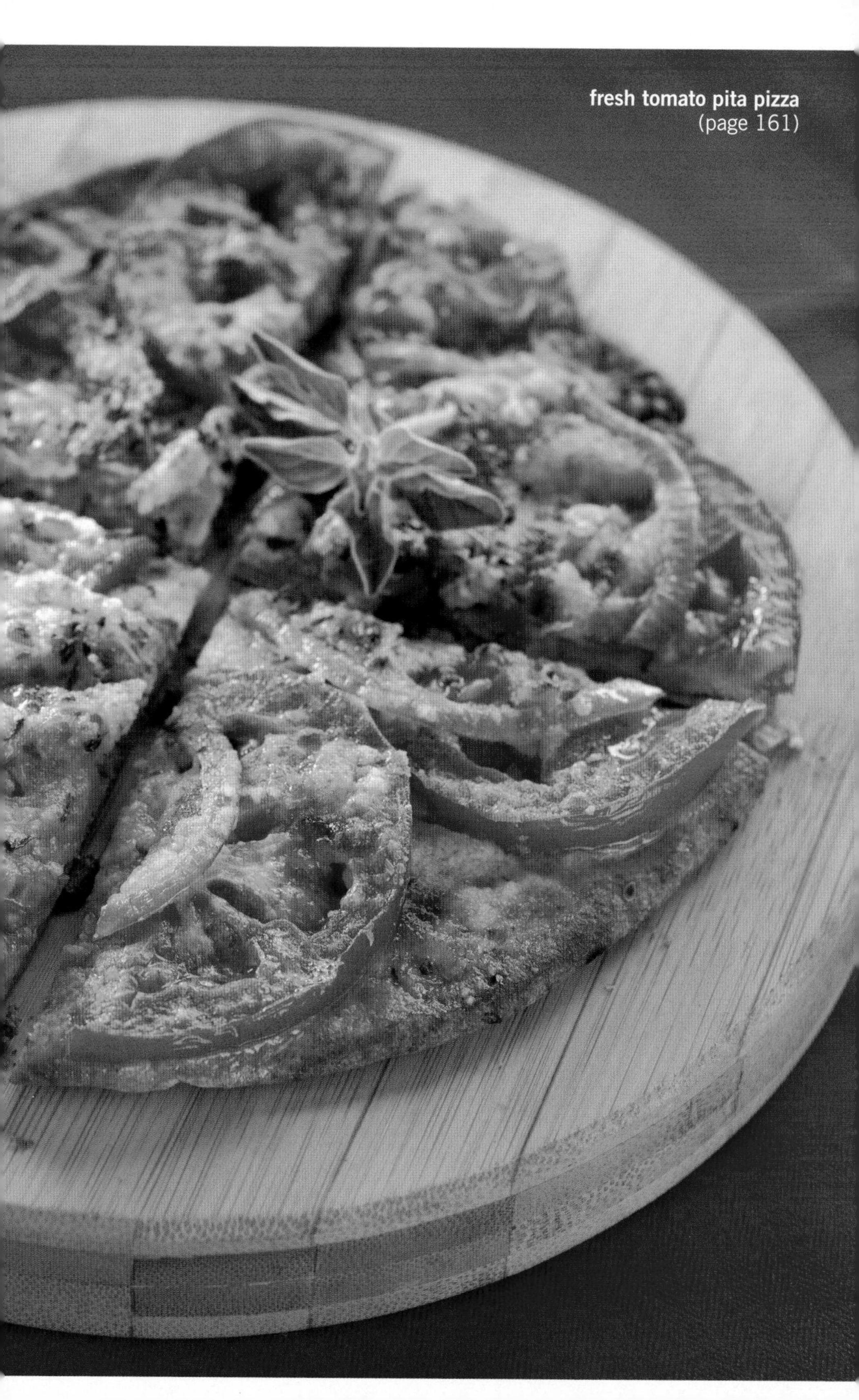

fresh tomato pita pizza
(page 161)

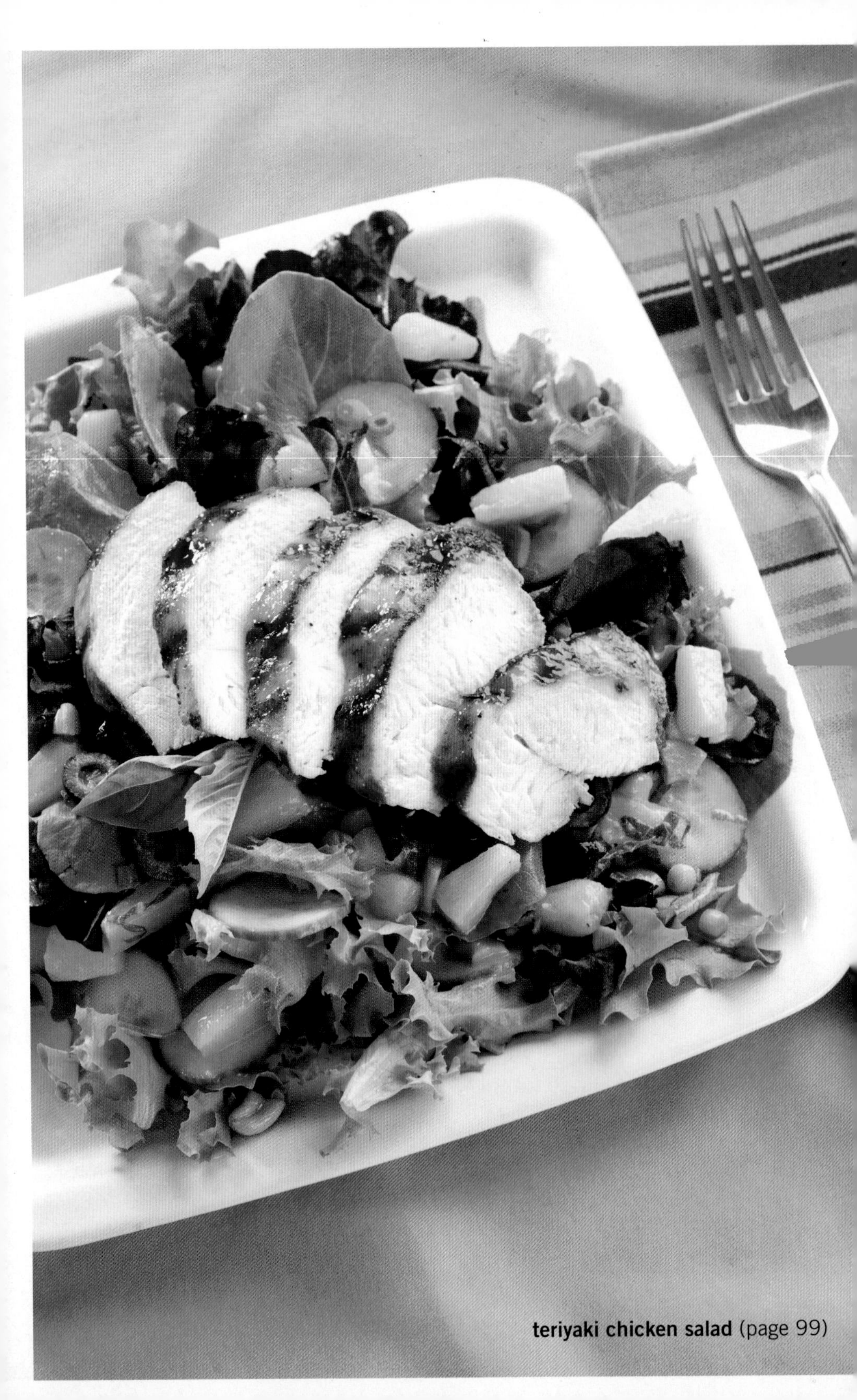

teriyaki chicken salad (page 99)

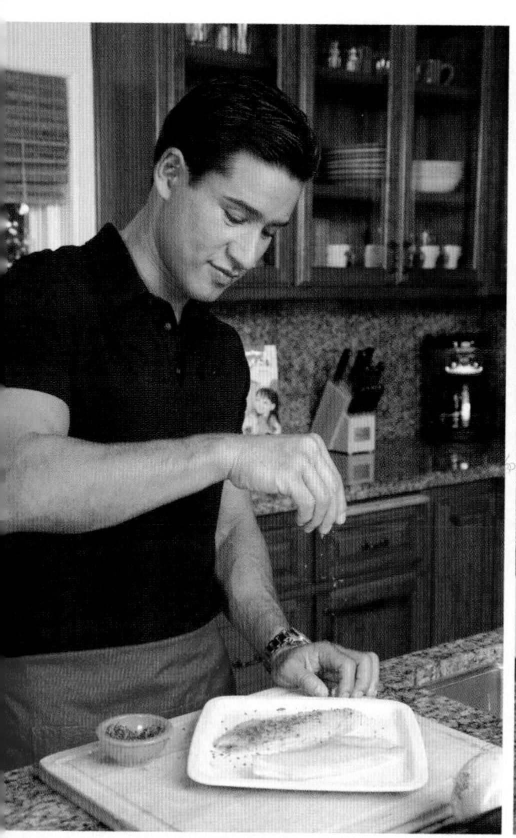

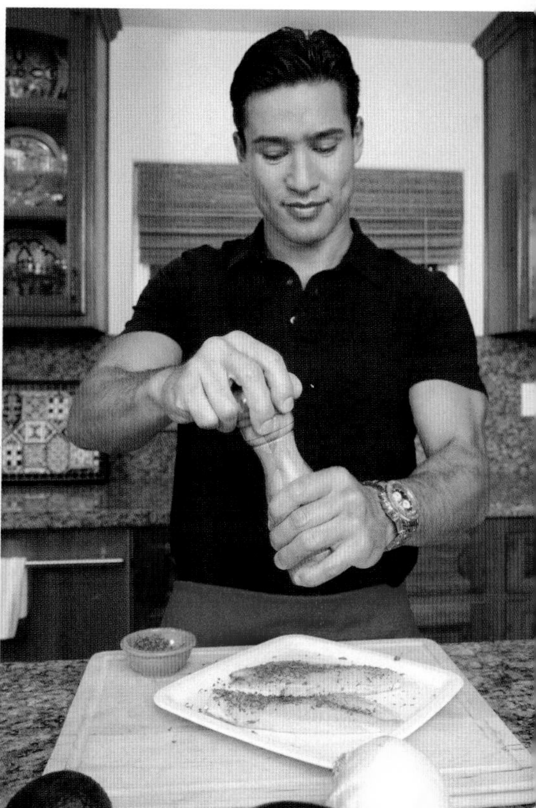

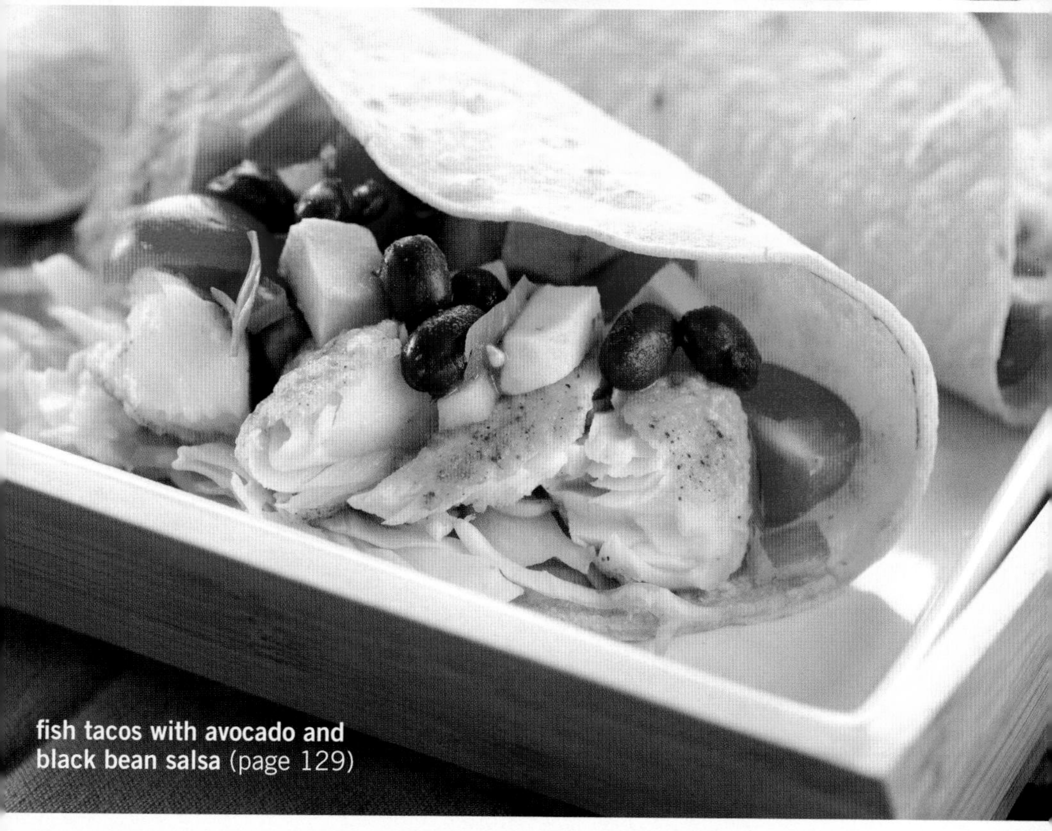

fish tacos with avocado and black bean salsa (page 129)

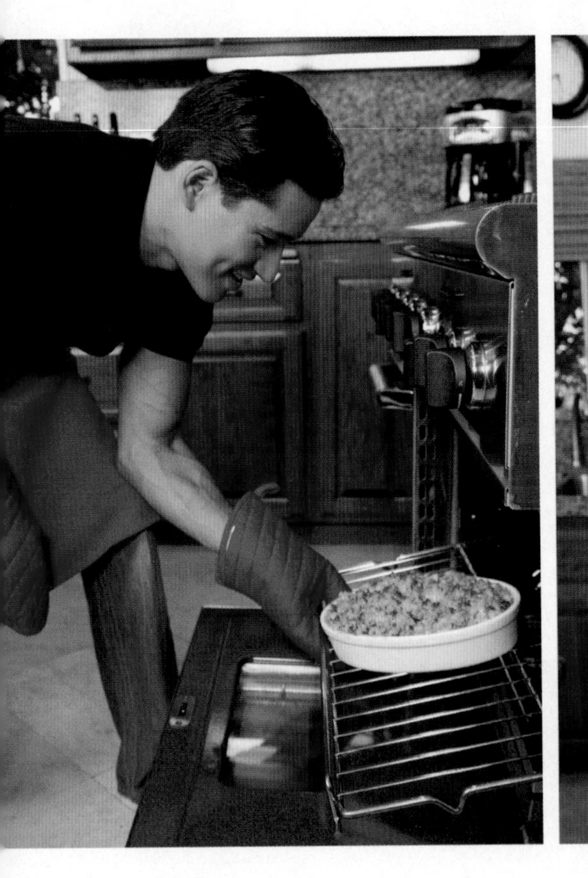

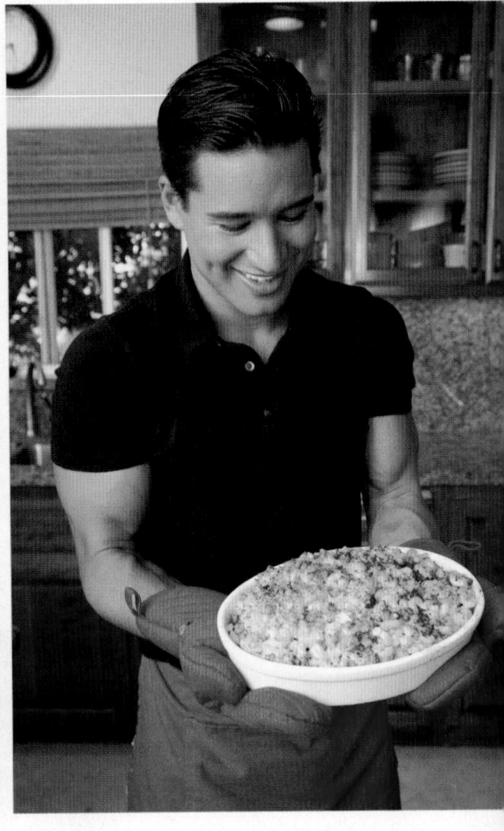

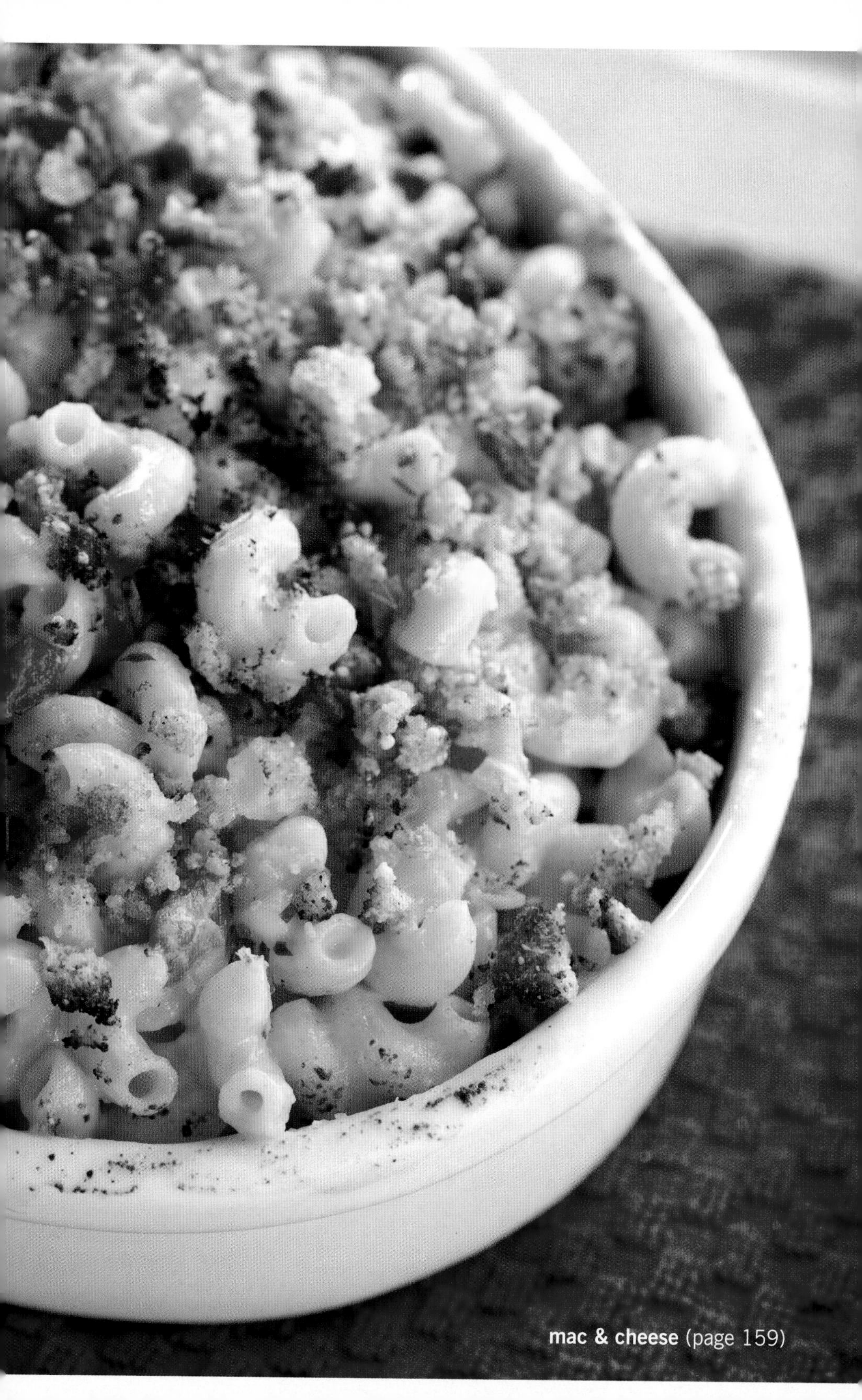
mac & cheese (page 159)

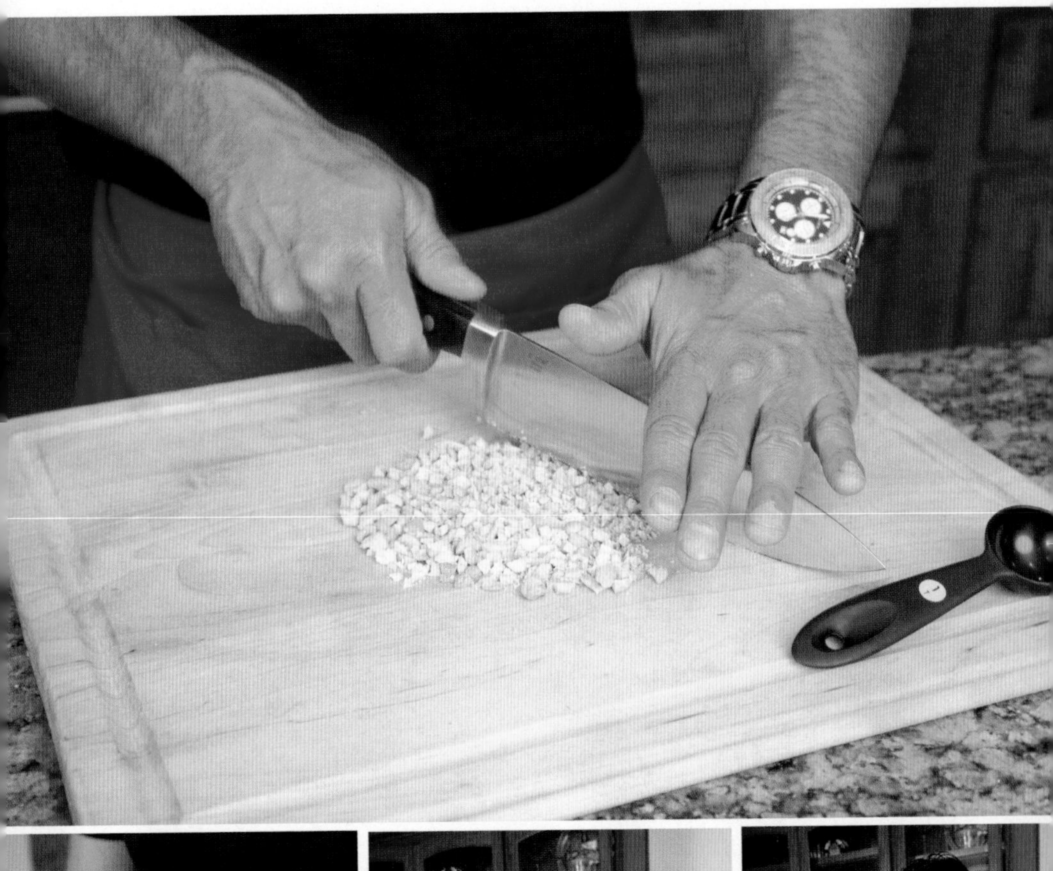

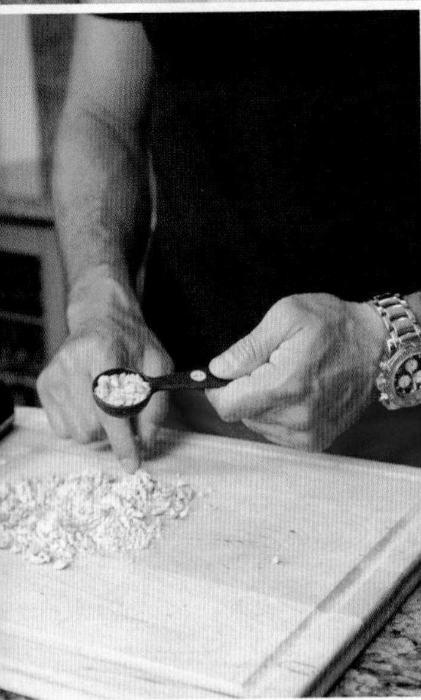

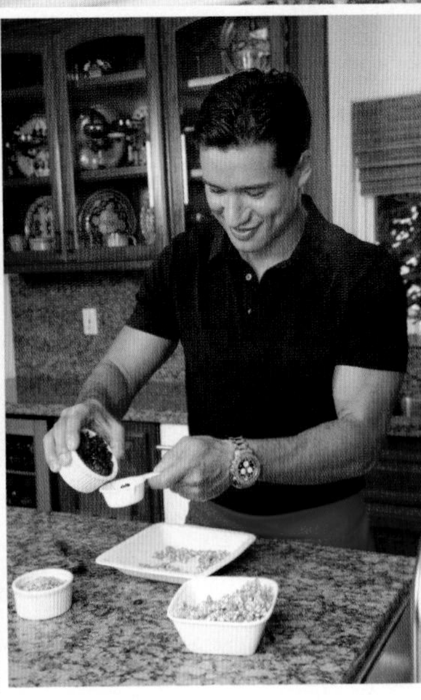

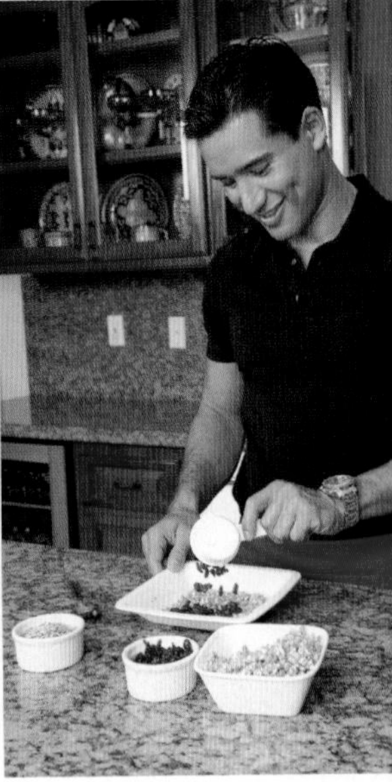

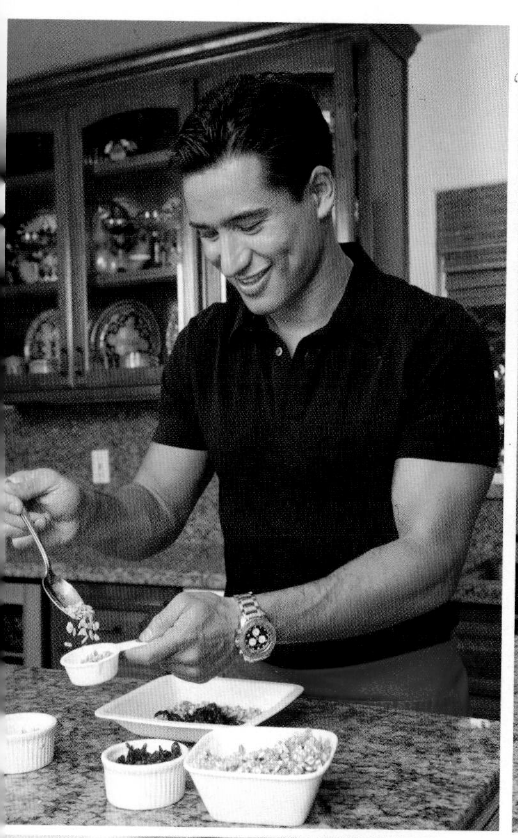

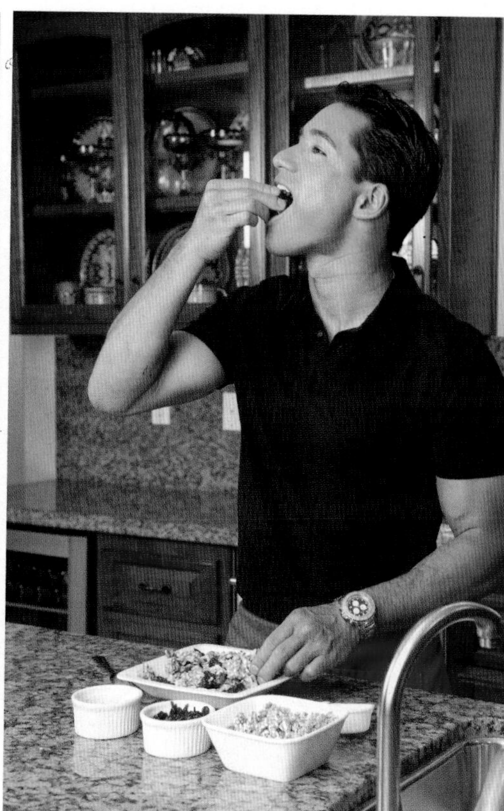

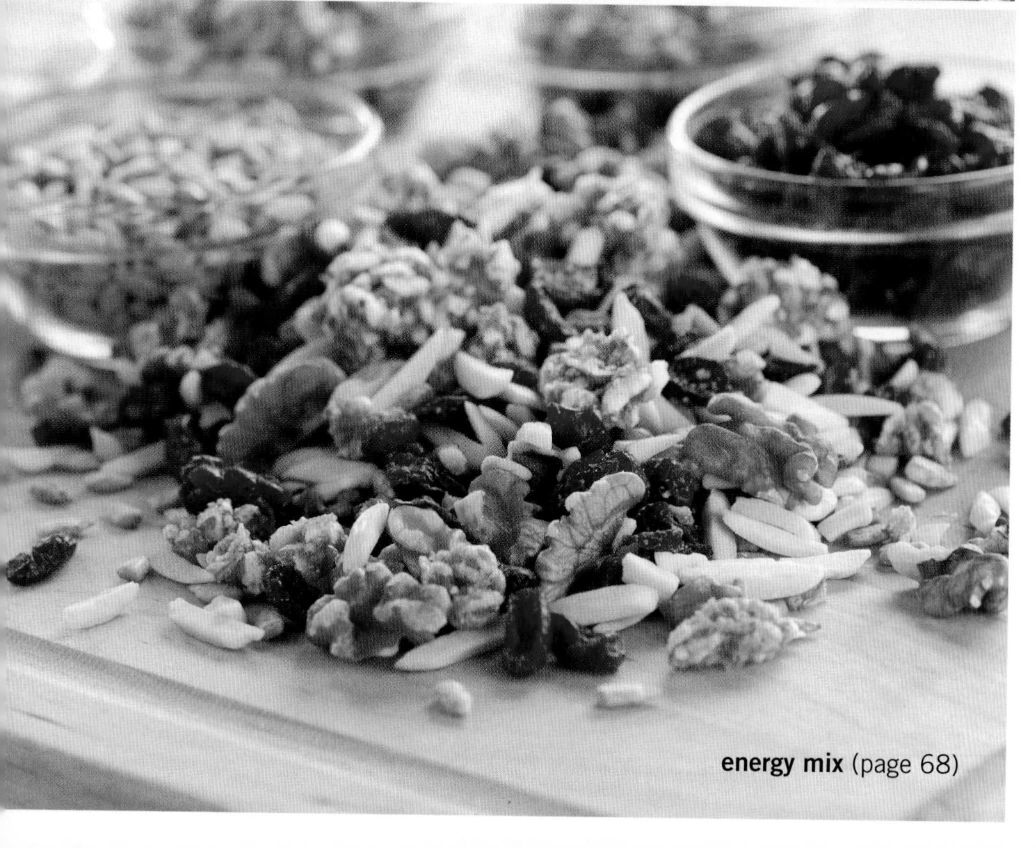

energy mix (page 68)

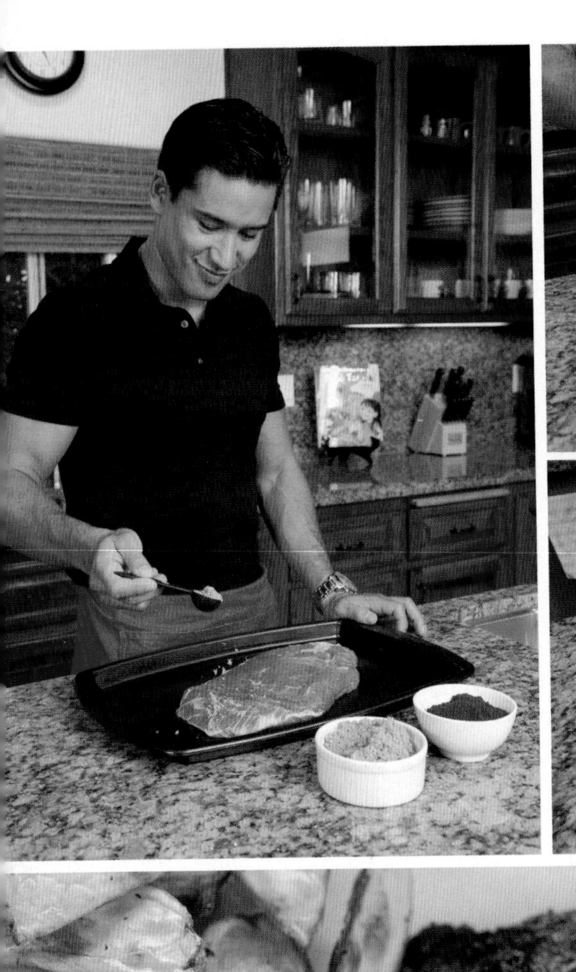

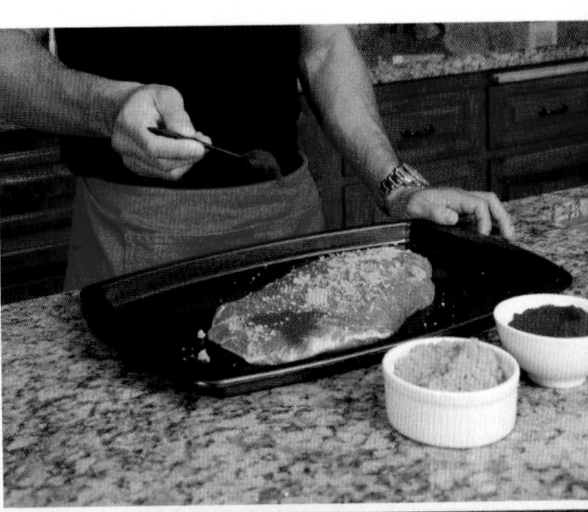

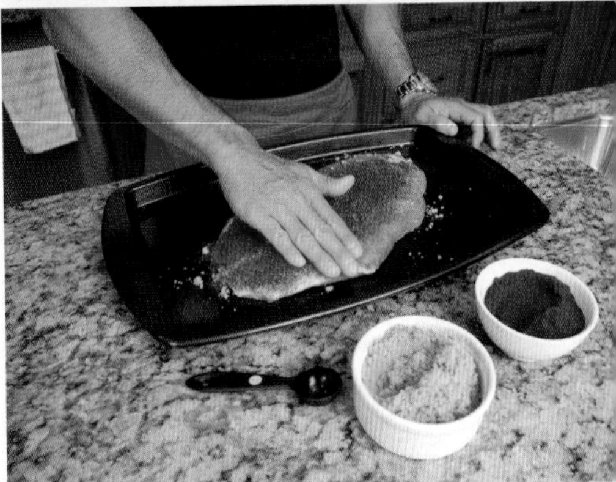

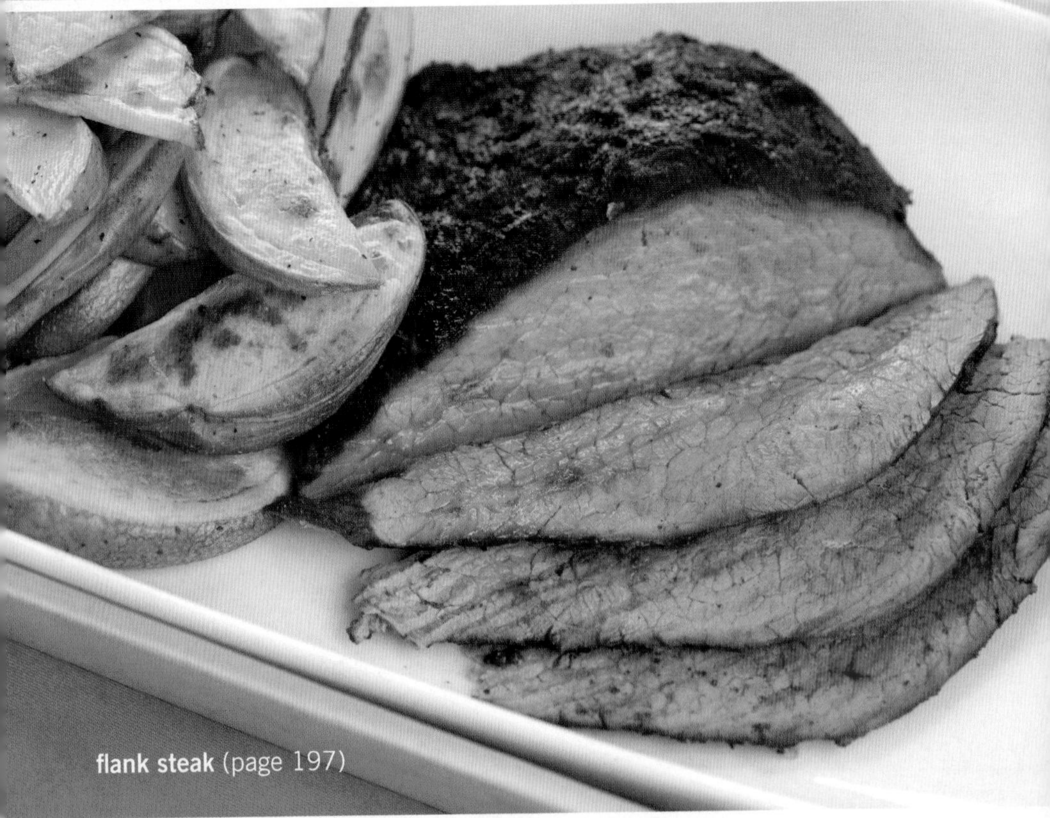

flank steak (page 197)

SNACK 3

▶ **1 granola bar (Kashi)**

Total Calories: 130 kcal
Total Fat: 5 g
Saturated Fat: 0.5 g
Total Carbohydrate: 20 g
Protein: 5 g
Sodium: 90 mg
Fiber: 4 g

NUTRIENT INTAKE:

55% carbs
14% protein
31% fat

DINNER

▶ **Tofu stir-fry**

Tofu Stir-Fry

SERVES: 1

** half of the tofu (about 3 oz) you cook here will be reserved for tomorrow's lunch*

7 oz (½ package) extra-firm tofu, cubed
1 tsp dark sesame oil
1 Tbsp reduced-sodium soy sauce
1 tsp rice vinegar
1 tsp hoisin sauce
1 Tbsp water
½ tsp cornstarch

1 tsp canola oil
½ tsp freshly grated ginger
1 cup chopped broccoli
1 cup shredded green cabbage
½ cup sliced carrots

1. Drain sliced tofu on a paper towel for 5 to 10 minutes.
2. In a small bowl combine sesame oil, soy sauce, vinegar, hoisin, and water. Pour 1 Tbsp of the sauce over tofu and toss to coat.
3. Add cornstarch to remaining sauce, stir to combine and set aside.
4. Heat canola oil in a nonstick skillet wok over medium-high heat.
5. Add tofu and cook for 6 or 7 minutes until golden. Transfer cooked tofu to a bowl (reserve ½ for lunch tomorrow).
6. Add ginger, remaining sauce, broccoli, carrots, and cabbage to skillet and cook for 5 minutes until broccoli is just tender.
7. Return tofu to pan, toss well, and serve.

A cholesterol-free vegetarian source of protein, tofu takes on the flavor of whatever you cook it with.

Sesame oil has wonderful flavor and a little goes a long way. A couple of teaspoons is all you need for an entire recipe.

Total Calories: 299 kcal
Total Fat: 15.5 g
Saturated Fat: 2 g
Total Carbohydrate: 25 g
Protein: 16 g
Sodium: 557 mg
Fiber: 8 g

NUTRIENT INTAKE:

46% carbs
18% protein
36% fat

SNACK 4 (OPTIONAL)

▸ Cran-Orange Ice Pop

SERVES: 4

1 cup cranberry juice cocktail
1 cup orange juice
Juice of ½ lemon (optional)

1. Combine juices in a bowl and mix.
2. Transfer to paper cups or popsicle molds and place in the freezer until solid (if using paper cups, place popsicle sticks into cups halfway through freezing).

Total Calories: 65 kcal
Total Fat: 0 g
Saturated Fat: 0 g
Total Carbohydrate: 16 g
Protein: 0 g
Sodium: 3 mg
Fiber: 0 g

NUTRIENT INTAKE:

95% carbs
3% protein
2% fat

NUTRITION FOR THE DAY

Total Calories: 1325 kcal
Total Fat: 43 g
Saturated Fat: 7 g
Total Carbohydrate: 166 g
Protein: 82 g
Sodium: 1379 mg
Fiber: 34 g

NUTRIENT INTAKE:

58% carbs
19% protein
23% fat

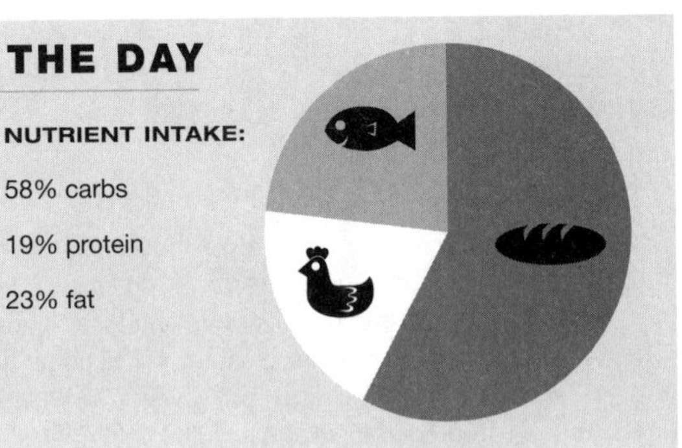

BREAKFAST

- **1 cup whole grain cereal (suggestions: Bran Flakes, Nature's Path Heirloom Flakes)**
- **¾ cup skim milk**
- **½ cup blueberries**

Total Calories: 257 kcal
Total Fat: 2.5 g
Saturated Fat: 0.5 g
Total Carbohydrate: 53 g
Protein: 12 g
Sodium: 79 mg
Fiber: 8 g

NUTRIENT INTAKE:

75% carbs
17% protein
8% fat

SNACK 1

- **1 hard-boiled egg**

Total Calories: 78 kcal
Total Fat: 5 g
Saturated Fat: 1.5 g
Total Carbohydrate: 1 g
Protein: 6 g
Sodium: 62 mg
Fiber: 0 g

NUTRIENT INTAKE:

3% carbs
33% protein
64% fat

LUNCH

- **Tofu Wrap**

1 whole wheat tortilla
3 oz tofu (from Tofu Stir-Fry, Day 2 dinner)
½ cup chopped lettuce or cabbage
2 Tbsp diced avocado with fresh lime juice to taste

Total Calories: 260 kcal
Total Fat: 10 g
Saturated Fat: 1 g
Total Carbohydrate: 27 g
Protein: 13 g
Sodium: 176 mg
Fiber: 5 g

NUTRIENT INTAKE:

45% carbs
21% protein
34% fat

SNACK 2

- 15 almonds

Total Calories: 104 kcal
Total Fat: 9 g
Saturated Fat: 1 g
Total Carbohydrate: 30 g
Protein: 11 g
Sodium: 175 mg
Fiber: 7 g

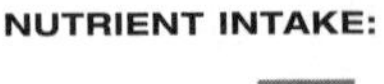
NUTRIENT INTAKE:

14% carbs
13% protein
73% fat

SNACK 3

- 1 medium pear
- 1 oz low fat cheddar cheese

Total Calories: 145 kcal
Total Fat: 2 g
Saturated Fat: 1 g
Total Carbohydrate: 26 g
Protein: 8 g
Sodium: 175 mg
Fiber: 5 g

NUTRIENT INTAKE:

68% carbs
19% protein
13% fat

DINNER

- 4 oz salmon roasted with 1 tsp olive oil, salt and pepper
- 1 medium baked sweet potato
- 1.5 cups mixed greens topped with 2 Tbsp light vinaigrette salad dressing

Total Calories: 360 kcal
Total Fat: 13.5 g
Saturated Fat: 2 g
Total Carbohydrate: 29 g
Protein: 30 g
Sodium: 597 mg
Fiber: 6 g

NUTRIENT INTAKE:

32% carbs
34% protein
34% fat

SNACK 4 (OPTIONAL)

▸ **1 large graham cracker (1 sheet)**

Total Calories: 59 kcal
Total Fat: 1 g
Saturated Fat: 0 g
Total Carbohydrate: 11 g
Protein: 1 g
Sodium: 85 mg
Fiber: 0 g

NUTRIENT INTAKE:

NUTRITION FOR THE DAY

Total Calories: 1263 kcal
Total Fat: 44 g
Saturated Fat: 8 g
Total Carbohydrate: 149 g
Protein: 74 g
Sodium: 1175 mg
Fiber: 26 g

NUTRIENT INTAKE:

43% carbs

21% protein

36% fat

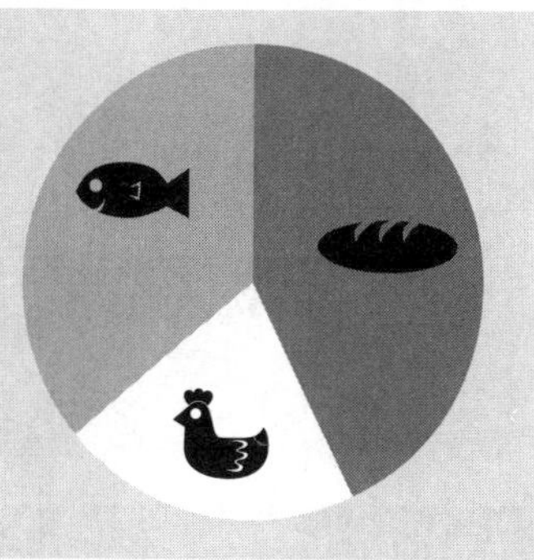

BREAKFAST

- 1 cup cooked steel-cut oatmeal topped with ½ cup sliced strawberries, 2 Tbsp chopped almonds, and 2 tsp maple syrup

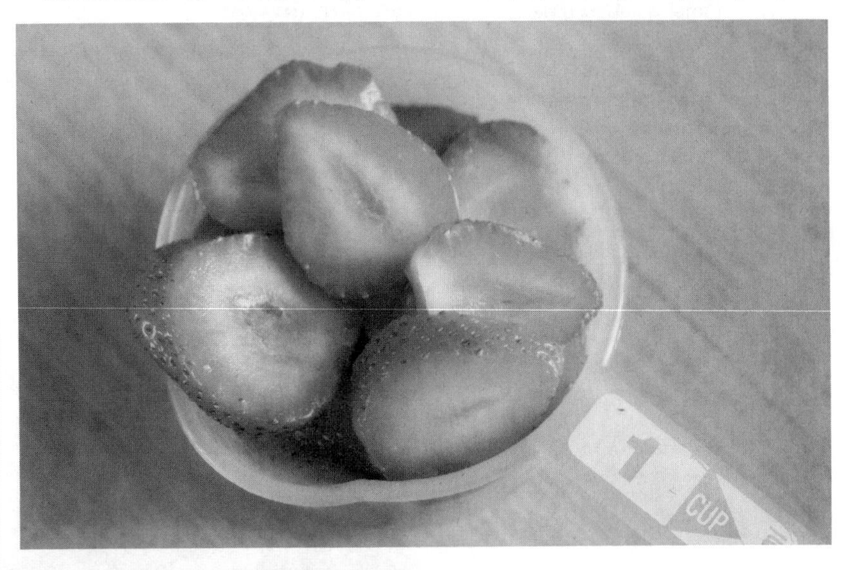

Another healthy oatmeal option, whole grain steel-cut oats have a different texture and the same amount of calories and fiber as rolled oats.

Total Calories: 291 kcal
Total Fat: 9.5 g
Saturated Fat: 1 g
Total Carbohydrate: 45 g
Protein: 8 g
Sodium: 2 mg
Fiber: 7 g

NUTRIENT INTAKE:

60% carbs
11% protein
29% fat

SNACK 1

- 6 oz nonfat fruit or vanilla yogurt

Total Calories: 130 kcal
Total Fat: 0 g
Saturated Fat: 0 g
Total Carbohydrate: 26 g
Protein: 6 g
Sodium: 105 mg
Fiber: 2 g

NUTRIENT INTAKE:

81% carbs
19% protein
0% fat

LUNCH

- **Salad with Tuna and Olives**

2 cups chopped lettuce
5 cherry tomatoes, halved
½ cup sliced cucumber
5 olives, sliced
¼ cup canned chickpeas, rinsed and drained
4 oz canned tuna (packed in water) mixed with 2 tsp light mayonnaise
Freshly squeezed lemon juice to taste

Total Calories: 283 kcal
Total Fat: 9 g
Saturated Fat: 0.5 g
Total Carbohydrate: 23 g
Protein: 31 g
Sodium: 887 mg
Fiber: 5 g

NUTRIENT INTAKE:
31% carbs
42% protein
27% fat

SNACK 2

- **1 medium pear**

Total Calories: 96 kcal
Total Fat: 0 g
Saturated Fat: 0 g
Total Carbohydrate: 26 g
Protein: 1 g
Sodium: 2 mg
Fiber: 5 g

NUTRIENT INTAKE:
96% carbs
2% protein
2% fat

SNACK 3

- **1 brown rice cake**
- **1 Tbsp natural peanut butter**

Total Calories: 140 kcal
Total Fat: 9 g
Saturated Fat: 1.5 g
Total Carbohydrate: 10 g
Protein: 4 g
Sodium: 17 mg
Fiber: 2 g

NUTRIENT INTAKE:
30% carbs
13% protein
57% fat

DINNER

- Spinach and sun dried tomato turkey burger
- 1 oz low fat cheddar cheese
- 1 cup steamed broccoli with lemon juice

Spinach and Sun Dried Tomato Turkey Burger

SERVES: 4

1 tsp olive oil
¼ cup finely chopped onion
2 Tbsp chopped sun dried tomatoes, packed in oil (drained)
1 cup baby spinach, roughly chopped
1 tsp kosher salt
½ tsp black pepper
1 lb ground turkey breast

1. Heat oil in a skillet over medium heat. Add onion and sauté for 2 to 3 minutes.
2. Add sun dried tomatoes, spinach, salt and pepper, and cook for an additional 1 to 2 minutes until spinach is just wilted. Set aside to cool.
3. Once spinach mixture is cooled, combine it with turkey and mix with clean hands until just combined—form into 4 burgers.
4. Preheat a grill, grill pan, or skillet and cook burgers for 6 or 7 minutes per side until cooked through.

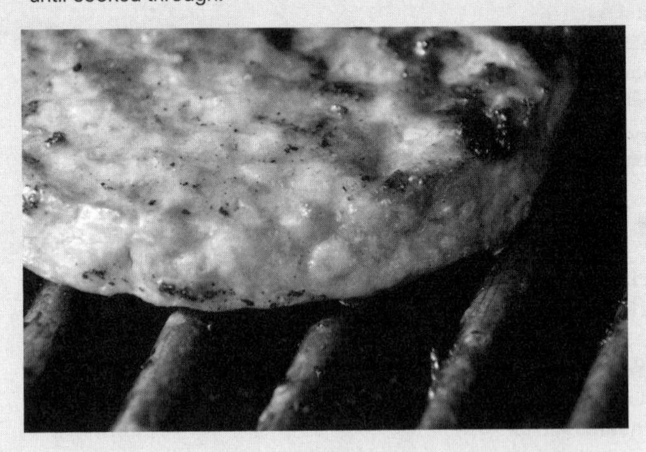

Total Calories: 248 kcal
Total Fat: 4.5 g
Saturated Fat: 1.5 g
Total Carbohydrate: 10 g
Protein: 41 g
Sodium: 655 mg
Fiber: 5 g

NUTRIENT INTAKE:

16% carbs
67% protein
17% fat

SNACK 4 (OPTIONAL)

▸ **10 almonds**

Total Calories: 69 kcal
Total Fat: 6 g
Saturated Fat: 0.5 g
Total Carbohydrate: 2 g
Protein: 3 g
Sodium: 0 mg
Fiber: 1 g

NUTRIENT INTAKE:

13% carbs 
14% protein
73% fat

NUTRITION FOR THE DAY

Total Calories: 1257 kcal
Total Fat: 38 g
Saturated Fat: 5 g
Total Carbohydrate: 142 g
Protein: 94 g
Sodium: 1669 mg
Fiber: 28 g

NUTRIENT INTAKE:

47% carbs
24% protein
29% fat

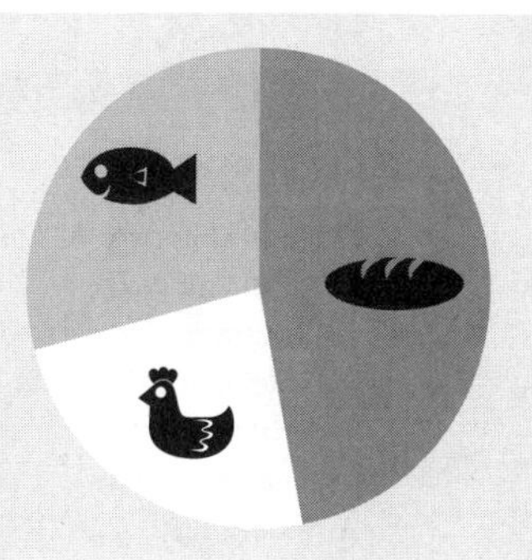

BREAKFAST

- **1 egg + 2 egg whites, scrambled with ½ cup chopped bell pepper and 2 Tbsp low fat cheddar cheese**
- **1 cup skim milk**

Total Calories: 235 kcal
Total Fat: 6.5 g
Saturated Fat: 2.5 g
Total Carbohydrate: 18 g
Protein: 26 g
Sodium: 370 mg
Fiber: 1 g

NUTRIENT INTAKE:

30% carbs
45% protein
25% fat

SNACK 1

- **1 medium orange**

Total Calories: 62 kcal
Total Fat: 0 g
Saturated Fat: 0 g
Total Carbohydrate: 15 g
Protein: 1 g
Sodium: 0 mg
Fiber: 3 g

NUTRIENT INTAKE:

91% carbs
7% protein
2% fat

LUNCH

- **Peanut Butter and Jelly**
  2 slices whole wheat bread
  1½ Tbsp natural peanut butter
  2 tsp natural fruit spread

Natural fruit spread is lower in sugar than jam and jelly.

Total Calories: 405 kcal
Total Fat: 16 g
Saturated Fat: 3 g
Total Carbohydrate: 51 g
Protein: 13 g
Sodium: 325 mg
Fiber: 8 g

NUTRIENT INTAKE:

51% carbs
14% protein
35% fat

SNACK 2

- 10 cherry tomatoes
- 2 Tbsp hummus

Total Calories: 77 kcal
Total Fat: 3 g
Saturated Fat: 0.5 g
Total Carbohydrate: 11 g
Protein: 4 g
Sodium: 115 mg
Fiber: 4 g

NUTRIENT INTAKE:

50% carbs
18% protein
32% fat

SNACK 3

- 1 granola bar (Kashi)

Total Calories: 130 kcal
Total Fat: 5 g
Saturated Fat: 0.5 g
Total Carbohydrate: 20 g
Protein: 5 g
Sodium: 90 mg
Fiber: 4 g

NUTRIENT INTAKE:

55% carbs
14% protein
31% fat

DINNER

- Fish tacos with avocado and black bean salsa

QUICK OPTION MEAL for fish tacos with avocado and black bean salsa < < < < < < < < < < <

- 5 oz broiled tilapia (prepared with 1 tsp olive oil and 1 tsp grill seasoning)
- 2 cups arugula topped with ½ cup chopped tomato and 2 tsp olive oil and lemon juice

Calories: 330 kcal
Total Fat: 18 g
Saturated Fat: 2.5 g
Total Carbohydrate: 5.5 g
Protein: 37 g
Sodium: 116 mg
Fiber: 2 g

Nutrition intake:

1% carbs
50% protein
49% fat

Tilapia is a lean white fish and requires very little cooking time.

Fish Tacos with Avocado and Black Bean Salsa

SERVES: 2

2 tilapia fillets (6 to 7 oz each)
¼ cup all-purpose flour
½ tsp salt
1 Tbsp chili powder
1 tsp canola oil

For the salsa:
½ cup diced avocado
½ cup cherry tomatoes, halved
1 Tbsp finely chopped onion
¼ cup canned black beans, rinsed and drained
1 Tbsp chopped cilantro
Juice of ½ a lime
¼ tsp kosher salt
Hot sauce to taste

4 corn tortillas, warmed
1 cup shredded green cabbage

1. Heat oil in a nonstick skillet over medium heat.
2. Season flour with salt and chili powder and flour fish on both sides (pat well to remove excess flour).
3. Cook fish in skillet for 4 to 5 minutes per side until golden.
4. When fish is cooked completely, transfer to a plate and break up into large pieces.
5. Combine salsa ingredients in a bowl and stir to combine.
6. Serve fish in corn tortillas topped with salsa and shredded cabbage.

Total Calories: 410 kcal
Total Fat: 9.5 g
Saturated Fat: 1 g
Total Carbohydrate: 38 g
Protein: 43 g
Sodium: 387 mg
Fiber: 9 g

NUTRIENT INTAKE:

37% carbs
42% protein
21% fat

SNACK 4 (OPTIONAL)

▸ **Cran-Orange Ice Pop**

Total Calories: 65 kcal
Total Fat: 0 g
Saturated Fat: 0 g
Total Carbohydrate: 16 g
Protein: 0 g
Sodium: 3 mg
Fiber: 0 g

NUTRIENT INTAKE:

95% carbs
3% protein
2% fat

NUTRITION FOR THE DAY

Total Calories: 1384 kcal
Total Fat: 40 g
Saturated Fat: 8 g
Total Carbohydrate: 169 g
Protein: 92 g
Sodium: 1291 mg
Fiber: 30 g

NUTRIENT INTAKE:

59% carbs
20% protein
21% fat

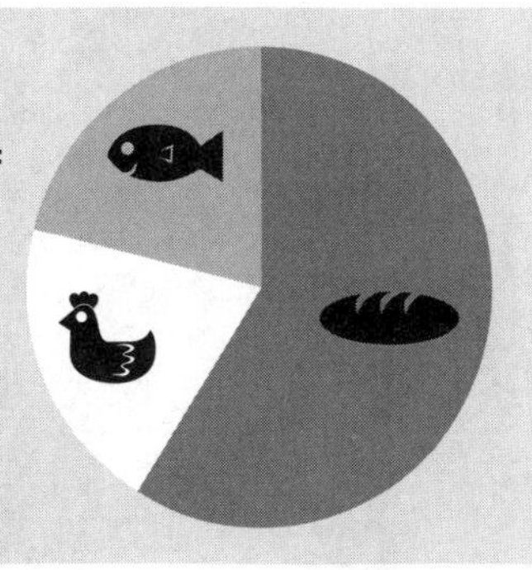

BREAKFAST

- 2 frozen whole grain waffles, toasted, topped with 2 tsp natural peanut butter
- ½ cup blueberries

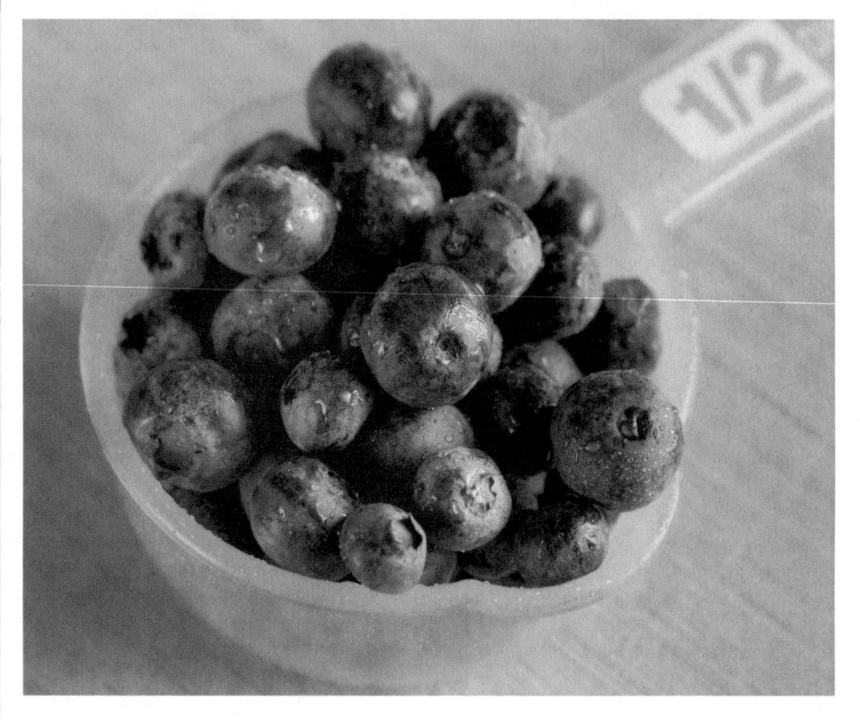

Total Calories: 181 kcal
Total Fat: 7 g
Saturated Fat: 1 g
Total Carbohydrate: 27 g
Protein: 5 g
Sodium: 226 mg
Fiber: 4 g

NUTRIENT INTAKE:

55% carbs
11% protein
34% fat

SNACK 1

- 1 brown rice cake
- 2 Tbsp hummus

Total Calories: 81 kcal
Total Fat: 3 g
Saturated Fat: 0.5 g
Total Carbohydrate: 11 g
Protein: 3 g
Sodium: 135 mg
Fiber: 2 g

NUTRIENT INTAKE:

48% carbs
18% protein
34% fat

LUNCH

▸ Garden Salad with Avocado and Sun Dried Tomatoes

2 cups chopped lettuce
5 cherry tomatoes, halved
2 Tbsp diced avocado
1 Tbsp sun dried tomatoes, packed in oil, drained
½ cup canned chickpeas, rinsed and drained
1 tsp olive oil
2 tsp fresh lemon juice

Total Calories: 256 kcal
Total Fat: 10 g
Saturated Fat: 1 g
Total Carbohydrate: 37 g
Protein: 8 g
Sodium: 403 mg
Fiber: 9 g

NUTRIENT INTAKE:

54% carbs
13% protein
33% fat

SNACK 2

▸ 1 medium orange

Total Calories: 62 kcal
Total Fat: 0 g
Saturated Fat: 0 g
Total Carbohydrate: 15 g
Protein: 1 g
Sodium: 0 mg
Fiber: 3 g

NUTRIENT INTAKE:

90% carbs
7% protein
3% fat

SNACK 3

▸ 1 hard-boiled egg

Total Calories: 78 kcal
Total Fat: 5 g
Saturated Fat: 1.5 g
Total Carbohydrate: 1 g
Protein: 6 g
Sodium: 62 mg
Fiber: 0 g

NUTRIENT INTAKE:

7% carbs
33% protein
60% fat

DINNER

- **5 oz grilled chicken breast**
- **1 medium sweet potato, diced and roasted with 1 tsp olive oil, salt and pepper**
- **1 cup steamed spinach**

Total Calories: 387 kcal
Total Fat: 5.5 g
Saturated Fat: 1.5 g
Total Carbohydrate: 33 g
Protein: 51 g
Sodium: 302 mg
Fiber: 8 g

NUTRIENT INTAKE:

36% carbs
53% protein
15% fat

DESSERT

- **Berry Crisp**

Berry Crisp

SERVES: 4

Nonstick cooking spray
1½ cups blueberries
1½ cups sliced strawberries
1 tsp cornstarch
Juice of ½ a lemon
¼ tsp lemon zest
1 Tbsp sugar

For the topping:
1 Tbsp unsalted butter, cut into 8 pieces
1 Tbsp all-purpose flour
¼ cup rolled oats
1 Tbsp light brown sugar
¼ tsp kosher salt
¼ cup slivered almonds

4 Tbsp plain nonfat Greek yogurt

1. Preheat oven to 350°F.
2. Spray 4 ramekins with cooking spray and place on a baking sheet.
3. In a medium bowl, combine berries, cornstarch, lemon juice, zest, and sugar—toss gently and set aside.
4. In a separate bowl, combine the topping ingredients and mix well with a fork or clean hands.
5. Fill each ramekin with berry mixture and evenly distribute topping over each.
6. Bake for 30 minutes until golden and bubbly. Serve topped with yogurt.

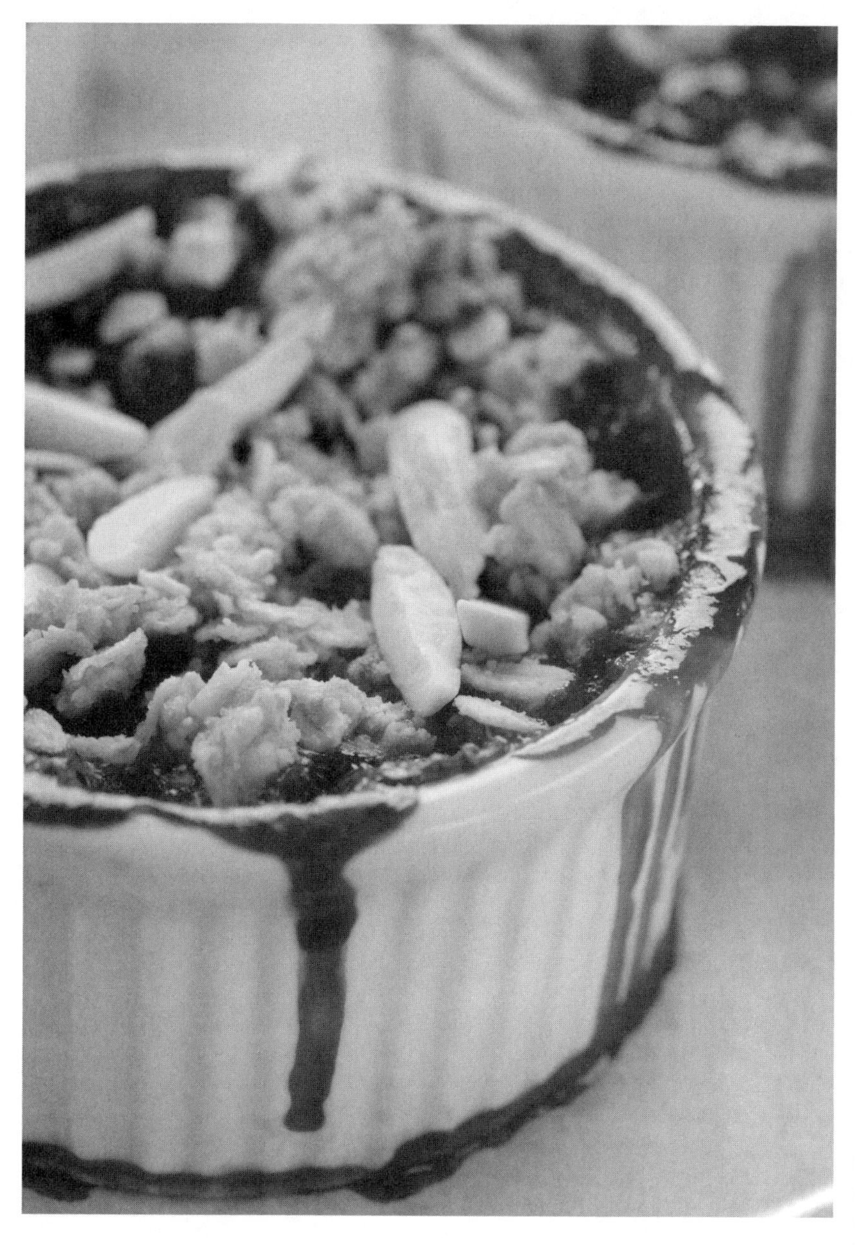

Total Calories: 181 kcal
Total Fat: 7 g
Saturated Fat: 2 g
Total Carbohydrate: 28 g
Protein: 4 g
Sodium: 77 mg
Fiber: 4 g

NUTRIENT INTAKE:

59% carbs

8% protein

33% fat

NUTRITION FOR THE DAY

Total Calories: 1225 kcal
Total Fat: 38 g
Saturated Fat: 8 g
Total Carbohydrate: 151 g
Protein: 80 g
Sodium: 1206 mg
Fiber: 30 g

NUTRIENT INTAKE:

50% carbs

20% protein

30% fat

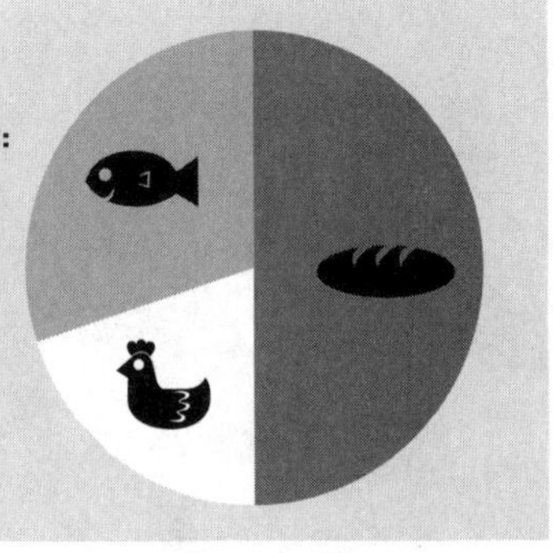

BREAKFAST

▸ **1 cup cooked steel-cut oatmeal topped with ½ cup sliced strawberries, 2 Tbsp chopped almonds, and 2 tsp maple syrup**

Total Calories: 291 kcal
Total Fat: 9.5 g
Saturated Fat: 1 g
Total Carbohydrate: 45 g
Protein: 8 g
Sodium: 2 mg
Fiber: 7 g

NUTRIENT INTAKE:

60% carbs
11% protein
29% fat

SNACK 1

▸ **1 medium orange**

Total Calories: 62 kcal
Total Fat: 0 g
Saturated Fat: 0 g
Total Carbohydrate: 15 g
Protein: 1 g
Sodium: 0 mg
Fiber: 3 g

NUTRIENT INTAKE:

91% carbs
7% protein
2% fat

LUNCH

▸ **Chicken and Rice Bowl**
3 oz grilled chicken breast
3 Tbsp diced avocado
2 Tbsp salsa
½ cup cooked brown rice

Total Calories: 302 kcal
Total Fat: 8 g
Saturated Fat: 1.5 g
Total Carbohydrate: 30 g
Protein: 30 g
Sodium: 268 mg
Fiber: 4 g

NUTRIENT INTAKE:

36% carbs
40% protein
24% fat

SNACK 2

- **6 oz nonfat fruit or vanilla yogurt**

Total Calories: 130 kcal
Total Fat: 0 g
Saturated Fat: 0 g
Total Carbohydrate: 26 g
Protein: 6 g
Sodium: 105 mg
Fiber: 2 g

NUTRIENT INTAKE:

81% carbs
19% protein
0% fat

SNACK 3

- **10 cherry tomatoes**
- **2 Tbsp hummus**

Total Calories: 77 kcal
Total Fat: 3 g
Saturated Fat: 0.5 g
Total Carbohydrate: 11 g
Protein: 4 g
Sodium: 115 mg
Fiber: 4 g

NUTRIENT INTAKE:

50% carbs
18% protein
32% fat

DINNER

- **4 oz broiled flank steak**
- **2 cups mixed greens topped with 2 Tbsp light vinaigrette salad dressing**

Flank steak is a lean, high-protein, flavorful, and affordable cut of beef.

Total Calories: 285 kcal
Total Fat: 13 g
Saturated Fat: 4.5 g
Total Carbohydrate: 6 g
Protein: 33 g
Sodium: 560 mg
Fiber: 3 g

NUTRIENT INTAKE:

9% carbs
48% protein
43% fat

SNACK 4 (OPTIONAL)

- 1 large graham cracker (1 sheet)

Total Calories: 59 kcal
Total Fat: 1 g
Saturated Fat: 0 g
Total Carbohydrate: 11 g
Protein: 1 g
Sodium: 85 mg
Fiber: 0 g

NUTRIENT INTAKE:

73% carbs

6% protein

21% fat

NUTRITION FOR THE DAY

Calories: 1207 kcal
Total Fat: 36 g
Saturated Fat: 8 g
Total Carbohydrate: 141 g
Protein: 83 g
Sodium: 1135 mg
Fiber: 24 g

NUTRIENT INTAKE:

57% carbs

21% protein

22% fat

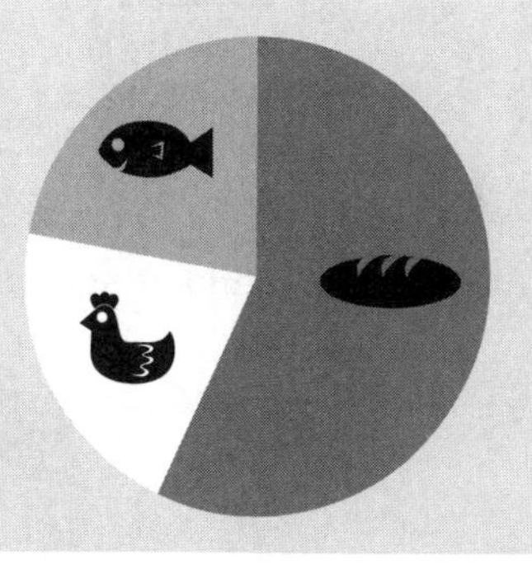

BREAKFAST

- ¾ cup nonfat cottage cheese topped with ½ cup sliced strawberries and 2 Tbsp chopped walnuts

Cottage cheese is a terrific source of protein and calcium.

Total Calories: 217 kcal
Total Fat: 10 g
Saturated Fat: 1 g
Total Carbohydrate: 11 g
Protein: 22 g
Sodium: 15 mg
Fiber: 3 g

NUTRIENT INTAKE:

20% carbs
39% protein
41% fat

SNACK 1

- ½ cup shelled edamame

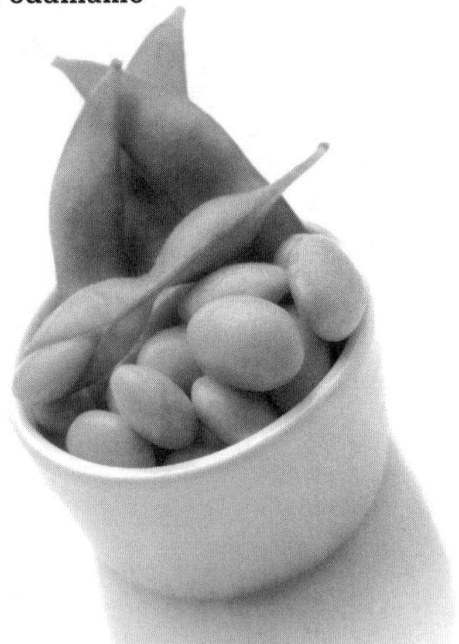

Total Calories: 90 kcal
Total Fat: 4 g
Saturated Fat: 1 g
Total Carbohydrate: 7 g
Protein: 8 g
Sodium: 7.5 mg
Fiber: 2 g

NUTRIENT INTAKE:

30% carbs
33% protein
37% fat

LUNCH

▸ **Turkey sandwich and small side salad**

Turkey Sandwich

1 whole wheat English muffin, toasted
3 oz low sodium turkey breast
3 slices tomato
2 tsp Dijon mustard

1½ cups mixed greens with 1 Tbsp low fat vinaigrette salad dressing

Total Calories: 282 kcal
Total Fat: 5 g
Saturated Fat: 0.5 g
Total Carbohydrate: 35 g
Protein: 27 g
Sodium: 1443 mg
Fiber: 7 g

NUTRIENT INTAKE:

48% carbs
37% protein
15% fat

SNACK 2

▸ **Fruit salad**

Fruit Salad

MAKES: 5 SERVINGS

1 ½ cups diced watermelon
1 ½ cups grapes, halved
1 ½ cups strawberries, halved
2 tangerines or 1 orange, peeled

Combine ingredients in a large bowl and toss. Store in an air tight container in the refrigerator for up to one week.

Total Calories: 80 kcal
Total Fat: 0 g
Saturated Fat: 0 g
Total Carbohydrate: 20 g
Protein: 1 g
Sodium: 280 mg
Fiber: 3 g

NUTRIENT INTAKE:

89% carbs
6% protein
5% fat

SNACK 3

- 1 part-skim mozzarella string cheese
- 1 oz whole wheat pretzels

Whole wheat pretzels are a great snack to get some extra fiber and to help curb hunger.

Total Calories: 183 kcal
Total Fat: 7 g
Saturated Fat: 3.5 g
Total Carbohydrate: 24 g
Protein: 10 g
Sodium: 278 mg
Fiber: 2 g

NUTRIENT INTAKE:

48% carbs
21% protein
31% fat

DINNER

- 4 oz grilled pork tenderloin
- ½ cup applesauce
- 1 cup steamed green beans topped with 1 tsp olive oil and lemon juice

Total Calories: 357 kcal
Total Fat: 12 g
Saturated Fat: 3 g
Total Carbohydrate: 23 g
Protein: 37 g
Sodium: 383 mg
Fiber: 6 g

NUTRIENT INTAKE:

27% carbs
42% protein
31% fat

SNACK 4 (OPTIONAL)

- 1 plum or tangerine

Total Calories: 30 kcal
Total Fat: 0 g
Saturated Fat: 0 g
Total Carbohydrate: 8 g
Protein: 0 g
Sodium: 0 mg
Fiber: 1 g

NUTRIENT INTAKE:

90% carbs
5% protein
5% fat

NUTRITION FOR THE DAY

Total Calories: 1239 kcal
Total Fat: 38 g
Saturated Fat: 9.5 g
Total Carbohydrate: 128 g
Protein: 105 g
Sodium: 2129 mg
Fiber: 24 g

NUTRIENT INTAKE:

43% carbs

30% protein

27% fat

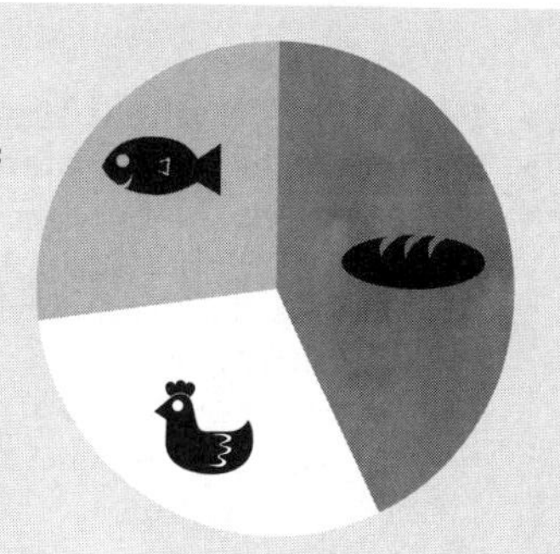

BREAKFAST

- 1 slice whole wheat bread, toasted
- 3 egg whites, scrambled
- 1 cup grapes

Total Calories: 223 kcal
Total Fat: 2 g
Saturated Fat: 0.5 g
Total Carbohydrate: 37 g
Protein: 15 g
Sodium: 316 mg
Fiber: 4 g

NUTRIENT INTAKE:

65% carbs
27% protein
8% fat

SNACK 1

- ½ cup shelled edamame

Total Calories: 90 kcal
Total Fat: 4 g
Saturated Fat: 1 g
Total Carbohydrate: 7 g
Protein: 8 g
Sodium: 7.5 mg
Fiber: 2 g

NUTRIENT INTAKE:

30% carbs
33% protein
37% fat

LUNCH

- 2 cups mixed greens
- Tuna and apples

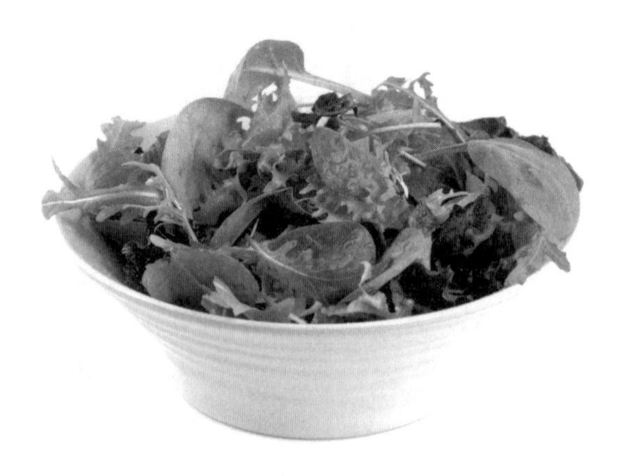

Tuna and Apples

SERVES: 1

5 oz can tuna, packed in water, drained
¼ cup chopped celery
1 Tbsp mayonnaise
½ cup diced apple
1 tsp honey
Black pepper to taste

Combine ingredients in a bowl and mix well.

It's okay to have small amounts of mayo here and there, just measure out those portions.

Total Calories: 309 kcal
Total Fat: 12.5 g
Saturated Fat: 1.5 g
Total Carbohydrate: 17 g
Protein: 34 g
Sodium: 745 mg
Fiber: 3 g

NUTRIENT INTAKE:

22% carbs
42% protein
36% fat

SNACK 2

▸ **1 medium banana**

Calories: 105 kcal
Total Fat: 0 g
Saturated Fat: 0 g
Total Carbohydrate: 27 g
Protein: 1 g
Sodium: 1 mg
Fiber: 3 g

NUTRIENT INTAKE:

92% carbs
4% protein
4% fat

SNACK 3

▸ **Energy mix (see recipe on page 68)**

Calories: 146 kcal
Total Fat: 12 g
Saturated Fat: 1 g
Total Carbohydrate: 8 g
Protein: 4 g
Sodium: 10 mg
Fiber: 2 g

NUTRIENT INTAKE:

40% carbs
33% protein
27% fat

DINNER

- 1 cup steamed zucchini
- Chicken enchilada

QUICK OPTION MEAL for chicken enchiladas < < < < < < < <

5 oz grilled chicken breast
1 medium sweet potato, diced, and roasted with 1 tsp olive oil, salt and pepper
1 cup steamed spinach

Total Calories: 387 kcal
Total Fat: 5.5 g
Saturated Fat: 1.5 g
Total Carbohydrate: 33 g
Protein: 51 g
Sodium: 302 mg
Fiber: 8 g

NUTRIENT INTAKE:

34% carbs
53% protein
13% fat

Chicken Enchiladas

SERVES: 3

6 corn tortillas
2 tsp olive oil
½ cup diced bell pepper
½ cup diced onion
½ tsp salt
½ tsp dried oregano
6 oz cooked chicken breast, shredded
2 Tbsp canned green chilies
1 cup mild salsa, divided
2 cups baby spinach
½ cup low fat shredded cheese (cheddar or Monterey Jack recommended)
Chopped scallions
Hot sauce (optional)
Nonstick cooking spray

1. Preheat oven to 375°F.
2. Wrap tortillas in aluminum foil and place in the oven to warm.
3. Heat oil in a large skillet over medium heat; add onions and peppers. Season with salt and oregano and sauté for 5 minutes.
4. Add chicken, green chilies, ½ cup salsa, and spinach and cook until spinach is wilted.
5. Remove tortillas from the oven and spray a 9 x 9 inch baking dish with non-stick cooking spray.

6. Place ¼ cup of chicken mixture in a tortilla, roll up and transfer to baking dish; repeat with remaining tortillas.
7. Top tortillas with remaining salsa and cheese and bake for 10 minutes until cheese is melted. Garnish with chopped scallions and serve with hot sauce, if desired.

Total Calories: 342 kcal
Total Fat: 10.5 g
Saturated Fat: 4 g
Total Carbohydrate: 36 g
Protein: 29 g
Sodium: 940 mg
Fiber: 8 g

NUTRIENT INTAKE:

40% carbs

33% protein

27% fat

SNACK 4 (OPTIONAL)

- **1 cup air-popped popcorn**

Total Calories: 31 kcal
Total Fat: 0 g
Saturated Fat: 0 g
Total Carbohydrate: 6 g
Protein: 1 g
Sodium: 1 mg
Fiber: 1 g

NUTRIENT INTAKE:

77% carbs

13% protein

10% fat

NUTRITION FOR THE DAY

Total Calories: 1247 kcal
Total Fat: 42 g
Saturated Fat: 8 g
Total Carbohydrate: 137 g
Protein: 92 g
Sodium: 2020 mg
Fiber: 24 g

NUTRIENT INTAKE:

49% carbs

23% protein

28% fat

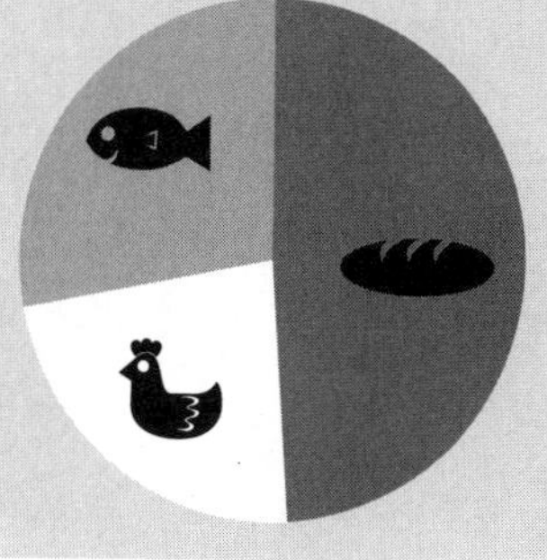

BREAKFAST

- **1 cup whole grain cereal (suggestions: Bran Flakes, Nature's Path Heirloom Flakes)**
- **¾ cup skim milk**
- **½ banana, sliced (* freeze other half for snack # 4)**

> Choose nonfat milk and yogurt to save calories and get all the protein and calcium of regular dairy.

Total Calories: 268 kcal
Total Fat: 2 g
Saturated Fat: 1 g
Total Carbohydrate: 56 g
Protein: 12 g
Sodium: 79 mg
Fiber: 8 g

NUTRIENT INTAKE:

76% carbs
17% protein
7% fat

SNACK 1

- **Fruit salad**

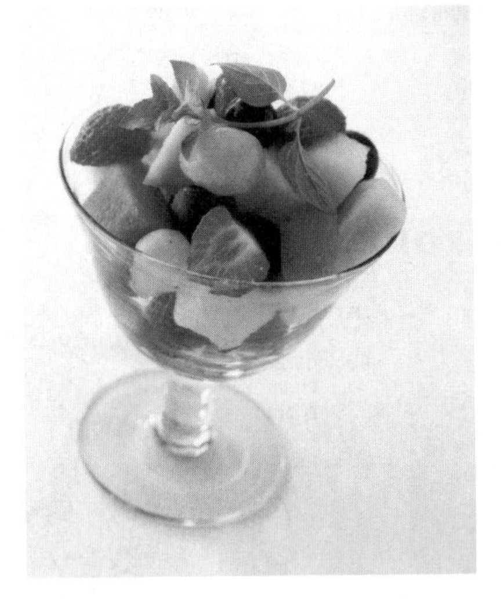

Total Calories: 80 kcal
Total Fat: 0 g
Saturated Fat: 0 g
Total Carbohydrate: 20 g
Protein: 1 g
Sodium: 280 mg
Fiber: 3 g

NUTRIENT INTAKE:

89% carbs
6% protein
5% fat

LUNCH

- 1½ cups low sodium lentil or black bean soup (Amy's)
- 2 cups mixed greens topped with 2 tsp olive oil and 2 tsp balsamic vinegar

Total Calories: 371 kcal
Total Fat: 19.5 g
Saturated Fat: 2.5 g
Total Carbohydrate: 40 g
Protein: 12 g
Sodium: 537 mg
Fiber: 12 g

NUTRIENT INTAKE:

42% carbs
12% protein
46% fat

SNACK 2

- 2 oz low sodium turkey breast, rolled up

Total Calories: 60 kcal
Total Fat: 1 g
Saturated Fat: 0 g
Total Carbohydrate: 0 g
Protein: 13 g
Sodium: 350 mg
Fiber: 0 g

NUTRIENT INTAKE:

0% carbs
85% protein
15% fat

SNACK 3

- 1 part-skim mozzarella string cheese

Total Calories: 80 kcal
Total Fat: 6 g
Saturated Fat: 3.5 g
Total Carbohydrate: 1 g
Protein: 7 g
Sodium: 220 mg
Fiber: 0 g

NUTRIENT INTAKE:

5% carbs
33% protein
62% fat

DINNER

- 5 oz grilled fish (such as mahi mahi or cod)
- 1 cup sautéed Swiss chard with 1 tsp olive oil and 1 tsp lemon juice
- ⅓ cup cooked quinoa (* make extra quinoa for tomorrow night's dinner)

One cup of Swiss chard contains over 700% of your daily vitamin K needs.

Total Calories: 296 kcal
Total Fat: 7.5 g
Saturated Fat: 1 g
Total Carbohydrate: 20 g
Protein: 39 g
Sodium: 476 mg
Fiber: 5 g

NUTRIENT INTAKE:

26% carbs
52% protein
22% fat

SNACK 4 (OPTIONAL)

▸ ½ frozen banana

Total Calories: 53 kcal
Total Fat: 0 g
Saturated Fat: 0 g
Total Carbohydrate: 13 g
Protein: 1 g
Sodium: 1 mg
Fiber: 2 g

NUTRIENT INTAKE:

93% carbs
4% protein
3% fat

NUTRITION FOR THE DAY

Total Calories: 1207 kcal
Total Fat: 37 g
Saturated Fat: 8 g
Total Carbohydrate: 151 g
Protein: 85 g
Sodium: 1665 mg
Fiber: 29 g

NUTRIENT INTAKE:

47% carbs
30% protein
23% fat

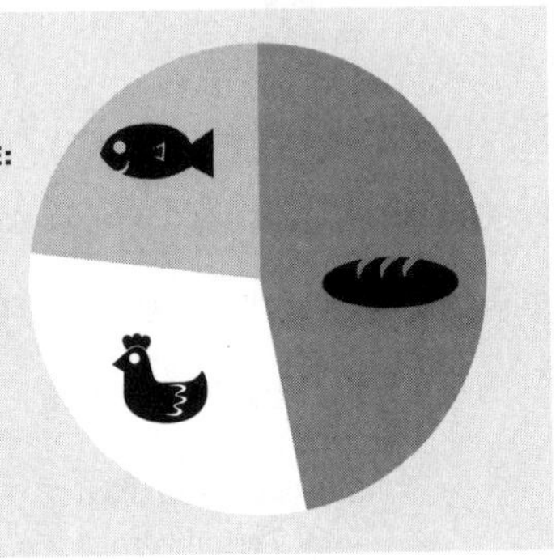

BREAKFAST

- **1 egg + 2 egg whites scrambled with ¼ cup baby spinach and ¼ cup chopped bell pepper**
- **½ whole wheat English muffin, toasted**

Total Calories: 255 kcal
Total Fat: 6.5 g
Saturated Fat: 2 g
Total Carbohydrate: 30 g
Protein: 20 g
Sodium: 612 mg
Fiber: 6 g

NUTRIENT INTAKE:

47% carbs
31% protein
22% fat

SNACK 1

- **Fruit salad**

Total Calories: 80 kcal
Total Fat: 0 g
Saturated Fat: 0 g
Total Carbohydrate: 20 g
Protein: 1 g
Sodium: 280 mg
Fiber: 3 g

NUTRIENT INTAKE:

88% carbs
7% protein
5% fat

LUNCH

- **½ Peanut Butter and Jelly Sandwich**
  1 slice whole wheat bread
  1 Tbsp natural peanut butter
  1 tsp natural fruit spread

Total Calories: 229 kcal
Total Fat: 10 g
Saturated Fat: 2 g
Total Carbohydrate: 26 g
Protein: 8 g
Sodium: 166 mg
Fiber: 5 g

NUTRIENT INTAKE:

44% carbs
14% protein
42% fat

SNACK 2

- ½ cup shelled edamame

Total Calories: 90 kcal
Total Fat: 4 g
Saturated Fat: 1 g
Total Carbohydrate: 7 g
Protein: 8 g
Sodium: 7.5 mg
Fiber: 2 g

NUTRIENT INTAKE:

30% carbs
33% protein
37% fat

SNACK 3

- ½ cup nonfat cottage cheese
- 1 Tbsp chopped walnuts

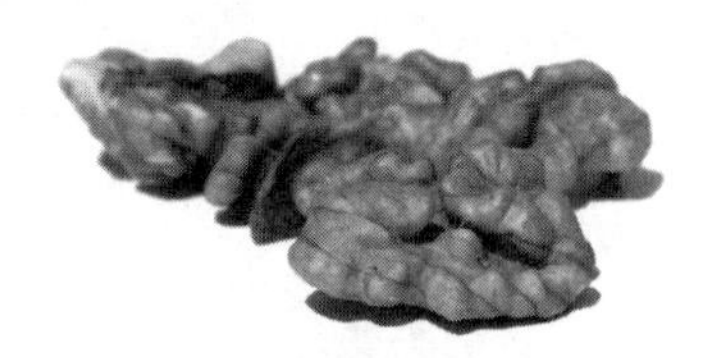

Total Calories: 128 kcal
Total Fat: 5 g
Saturated Fat: 0.5 g
Total Carbohydrate: 5 g
Protein: 16 g
Sodium: 380 mg
Fiber: 1 g

NUTRIENT INTAKE:

16% carbs
51% protein
33% fat

DINNER

- Quinoa stuffed peppers (recipe on page 78)

Total Calories: 427 kcal
Total Fat: 16 g
Saturated Fat: 4 g
Total Carbohydrate: 58 g
Protein: 20 g
Sodium: 255 mg
Fiber: 13 g

NUTRIENT INTAKE:

51% carbs
18% protein
31% fat

SNACK 4 (OPTIONAL)

- **1 plum or tangerine**

Total Calories: 30 kcal
Total Fat: 0 g
Saturated Fat: 0 g
Total Carbohydrate: 8 g
Protein: 0 g
Sodium: 0 mg
Fiber: 1 g

NUTRIENT INTAKE:

90% carbs
5% protein
5% fat

NUTRITION FOR THE DAY

Total Calories: 1239 kcal
Total Fat: 42 g
Saturated Fat: 9 g
Total Carbohydrate: 154 g
Protein: 73 g
Sodium: 1423 mg
Fiber: 29 g

NUTRIENT INTAKE:

52% carbs
23% protein
25% fat

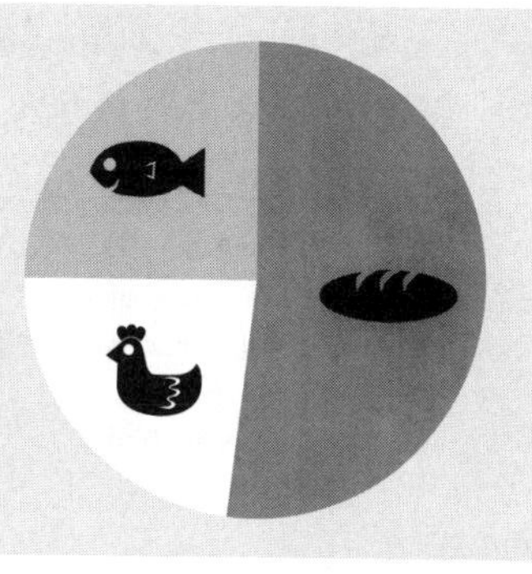

BREAKFAST

▸ **1 cup cooked oatmeal topped with 2 tsp honey and ½ cup sliced strawberries**

Total Calories: 219 kcal
Total Fat: 2.5 g
Saturated Fat: 0 g
Total Carbohydrate: 44 g
Protein: 7 g
Sodium: 4 mg
Fiber: 6 g

NUTRIENT INTAKE:

78% carbs
12% protein
10% fat

SNACK 1

▸ **Energy mix (see recipe on page 68)**

Total Calories: 146 kcal
Total Fat: 12 g
Saturated Fat: 1 g
Total Carbohydrate: 8 g
Protein: 4 g
Sodium: 10 mg
Fiber: 2 g

NUTRIENT INTAKE:

20% carbs
11% protein
69% fat

LUNCH

▸ **Spinach Salad with Grapes and Grilled Chicken**

2 cups baby spinach
½ cup sliced cucumber
¼ cup grapes, halved
3 oz grilled chicken breast, sliced
1 Tbsp white wine vinegar
2 tsp extra-virgin olive oil

Total Calories: 282 kcal
Total Fat: 12 g
Saturated Fat: 2 g
Total Carbohydrate: 13 g
Protein: 30 g
Sodium: 157 mg
Fiber: 3 g

NUTRIENT INTAKE:

19% carbs
42% protein
39% fat

SNACK 2

- 1 medium apple

Total Calories: 72 kcal
Total Fat: 0 g
Saturated Fat: 0 g
Total Carbohydrate: 19 g
Protein: 0 g
Sodium: 1 mg
Fiber: 0 g

NUTRIENT INTAKE:

96% carbs
3% protein
1% fat

SNACK 3

- 2 oz low sodium turkey breast
- 1 oz whole wheat pretzels

Total Calories: 163 kcal
Total Fat: 2 g
Saturated Fat: 0 g
Total Carbohydrate: 23 g
Protein: 16 g
Sodium: 408 mg
Fiber: 2 g

NUTRIENT INTAKE:

53% carbs
38% protein
9% fat

DINNER

- Tomato and Swiss omelet (see recipe on page 104)
- 1 slice whole grain bread, toasted
- 1 cup sliced cucumber topped with 2 Tbsp light vinaigrette salad dressing

Total Calories: 338 kcal
Total Fat: 12 g
Saturated Fat: 3.5 g
Total Carbohydrate: 30 g
Protein: 27 g
Sodium: 878 mg
Fiber: 4 g

NUTRIENT INTAKE:

35% carbs
32% protein
33% fat

SNACK 4 (OPTIONAL)

▸ **1 cup air-popped popcorn**

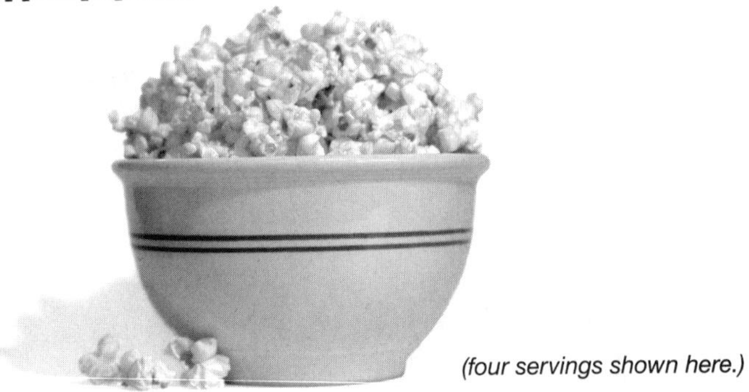

(four servings shown here.)

Total Calories: 31 kcal
Total Fat: 0 g
Saturated Fat: 0 g
Total Carbohydrate: 6 g
Protein: 1 g
Sodium: 1 mg
Fiber: 1 g

NUTRIENT INTAKE:

77% carbs
13% protein
10% fat

NUTRITION FOR THE DAY

Total Calories: 1250 kcal
Total Fat: 41.5 g
Saturated Fat: 7 g
Total Carbohydrate: 143 g
Protein: 85 g
Sodium: 1458 mg
Fiber: 22 g

NUTRIENT INTAKE:

54% carbs
22% protein
24% fat

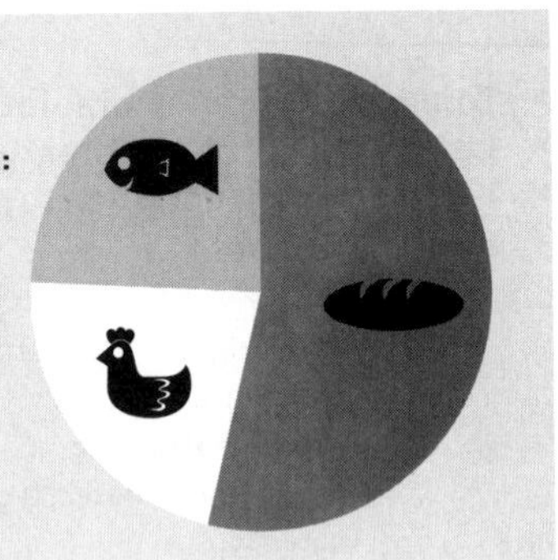

BREAKFAST

- **1 cup whole grain cereal (suggestions: Bran Flakes, Nature's Path Heirloom Flakes)**
- **¾ cup skim milk**
- **½ banana, sliced (* freeze other half for snack # 4)**

Total Calories: 268 kcal
Total Fat: 2 g
Saturated Fat: 1 g
Total Carbohydrate: 56 g
Protein: 12 g
Sodium: 79 mg
Fiber: 8 g

NUTRIENT INTAKE:

76% carbs
17% protein
7% fat

SNACK 1

- **½ cup applesauce**
- **½ cup nonfat cottage cheese**

Total Calories: 130 kcal
Total Fat: 0 g
Saturated Fat: 0 g
Total Carbohydrate: 18 g
Protein: 15 g
Sodium: 380 mg
Fiber: 1 g

NUTRIENT INTAKE:

55% carbs
45% protein
0% fat

LUNCH

- **Green Salad with Grilled Chicken**

2 cups mixed greens
½ cup sliced cucumber
¼ cup sliced red onion
3 oz grilled chicken breast, sliced
1 Tbsp sunflower seeds
1 Tbsp balsamic vinegar
2 tsp extra-virgin olive oil

Total Calories: 322 kcal
Total Fat: 16.5 g
Saturated Fat: 2.5 g
Total Carbohydrate: 14 g
Protein: 30 g
Sodium: 97 mg
Fiber: 4 g

NUTRIENT INTAKE:

17% carbs
37% protein
46% fat

SNACK 2

▸ **1 tangerine**

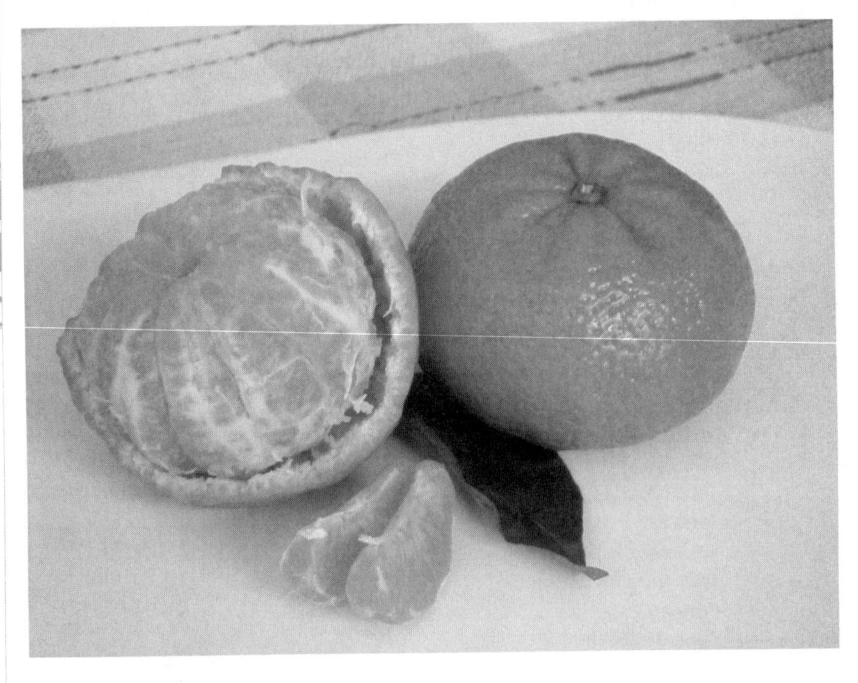

Total Calories: 45 kcal
Total Fat: 0 g
Saturated Fat: 0 g
Total Carbohydrate: 11 g
Protein: 1 g
Sodium: 2 mg
Fiber: 2 g

NUTRIENT INTAKE:

90% carbs
5% protein
5% fat

SNACK 3

▸ **2 oz low sodium turkey breast**

Total Calories: 60 kcal
Total Fat: 1 g
Saturated Fat: 0 g
Total Carbohydrate: 0 g
Protein: 13 g
Sodium: 350 mg
Fiber: 0 g

NUTRIENT INTAKE:

0% carbs
85% protein
15% fat

DINNER

- ½ cup sliced cucumber
- Mac & Cheese

Mac & Cheese

SERVES: 6

1 pound whole grain elbow macaroni (like whole wheat, Barilla PLUS, or Tinkyada brown rice pasta)
1 Tbsp unsalted butter
½ cup diced onion
½ tsp kosher salt
½ tsp black pepper
½ tsp Worcestershire sauce
1 Tbsp all-purpose flour
1 cup low fat (1%) milk
2 Tbsp reduced fat cream cheese (Neufchatel cheese)
1 cup shredded cheddar cheese
Pinch ground nutmeg
1 cup chopped roasted red peppers
Nonstick cooking spray

1 slice whole wheat bread
2 Tbsp grated Parmesan cheese
1 tsp olive oil
1 clove garlic

Choose whole wheat pasta such as Barilla or Tinkyada brown rice pasta.

1. Preheat oven to 350°F.
2. Cook pasta according to package directions.
3. While pasta is cooking, melt butter in a large saucepan.
4. Add onion, salt, pepper, and Worcestershire sauce, and sauté for 5 minutes.
5. Sprinkle flour over onions and cook, stirring constantly for 1 minute.
6. Whisk in milk and simmer until thickened.
7. Stir in cream cheese, cheddar, and nutmeg and cook until cheese is melted—turn off heat.
8. Add drained pasta to cheese mixture along with roasted peppers and mix well.
9. Transfer to a baking dish sprayed with nonstick cooking spray.
10. For the topping, place bread, cheese, oil, and garlic in a food processor fitted with a steel blade; pulse until bread is in fine crumbs.
11. Sprinkle bread crumbs over pasta and bake for 10 minutes until golden.

Total Calories: 465 kcal
Total Fat: 16 g
Saturated Fat: 6.5 g
Total Carbohydrate: 61 g
Protein: 21 g
Sodium: 677 mg
Fiber: 12 g

NUTRIENT INTAKE:

51% carbs
18% protein
31% fat

SNACK 4 (OPTIONAL)

- ½ medium banana

Total Calories: 53 kcal
Total Fat: 0 g
Saturated Fat: 0 g
Total Carbohydrate: 13 g
Protein: 1 g
Sodium: 1 mg
Fiber: 2 g

NUTRIENT INTAKE:

93% carbs
4% protein
3% fat

NUTRITION FOR THE DAY

Total Calories: 1328 kcal
Total Fat: 36.5 g
Saturated Fat: 10 g
Total Carbohydrate: 169 g
Protein: 93 g
Sodium: 1584 mg
Fiber: 28 g

NUTRIENT INTAKE:

55% carbs
30% protein
15% fat

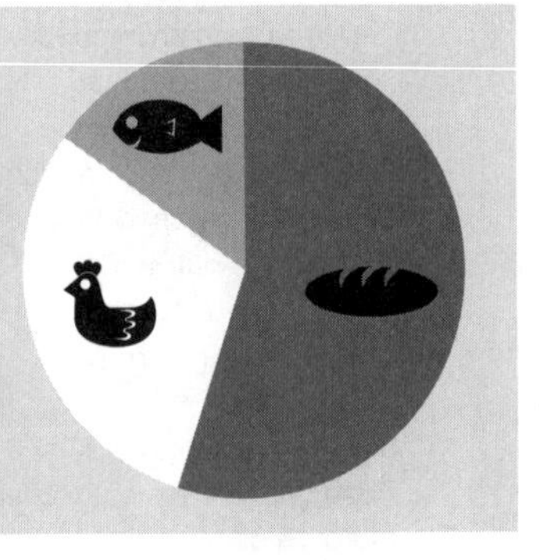

BREAKFAST

▸ **¾ cup nonfat cottage cheese topped with 1 cup sliced strawberries and 1 Tbsp sunflower seeds**

Total Calories: 166 kcal
Total Fat: 2 g
Saturated Fat: 0.5 g
Total Carbohydrate: 16 g
Protein: 21 g
Sodium: 16 mg
Fiber: 4 g

NUTRIENT INTAKE:

38% carbs
49% protein
13% fat

SNACK 1

▸ **Energy mix (recipe on page 68)**

Total Calories: 146 kcal
Total Fat: 12 g
Saturated Fat: 1 g
Total Carbohydrate: 8 g
Protein: 4 g
Sodium: 10 mg
Fiber: 2 g

NUTRIENT INTAKE:

20% carbs
11% protein
69% fat

LUNCH

▸ **Fresh tomato pita pizza**

Fresh Tomato Pita Pizza

SERVES: 1

1 whole wheat pita bread (6 inch)
4 slices tomato
1 clove minced garlic
3 thin rings red onion
¼ tsp dried oregano
Salt
2 Tbsp grated Parmesan cheese
1 tsp olive oil

Preheat oven to 400°F.

Place pita on a baking sheet lined with aluminum foil. Top pita with tomato, garlic, and onion; sprinkle with oregano, cheese, and a pinch of salt. Drizzle with oil and bake until golden and cheese is melted (about 10 to 12 minutes).

Total Calories: 290 kcal
Total Fat: 9 g
Saturated Fat: 2.5 g
Total Carbohydrate: 44 g
Protein: 11 g
Sodium: 499 mg
Fiber: 6 g

NUTRIENT INTAKE:

58% carbs
15% protein
27% fat

SNACK 2

- Fruit salad

Total Calories: 80 kcal
Total Fat: 0 g
Saturated Fat: 0 g
Total Carbohydrate: 20 g
Protein: 1 g
Sodium: 280 mg
Fiber: 3 g

NUTRIENT INTAKE:

62% carbs
14% protein
24% fat

SNACK 3

- 1 part-skim mozzarella string cheese
- 1 medium apple

Total Calories: 153 kcal
Total Fat: 6 g
Saturated Fat: 3.5 g
Total Carbohydrate: 20 g
Protein: 7 g
Sodium: 224 mg
Fiber: 3 g

NUTRIENT INTAKE:

48% carbs
18% protein
34% fat

DINNER

- 4 oz grilled chicken breast, prepared with 1 Tbsp BBQ sauce
- 1 cup steamed Swiss chard
- ½ cup cooked quinoa

Total Calories: 340 kcal
Total Fat: 6 g
Saturated Fat: 1 g
Total Carbohydrate: 29 g
Protein: 43 g
Sodium: 531 mg
Fiber: 6 g

NUTRIENT INTAKE:

34% carbs
50% protein
16% fat

DESSERT

- 1 oz dark chocolate

Total Calories: 146 kcal
Total Fat: 9 g
Saturated Fat: 5 g
Total Carbohydrate: 17 g
Protein: 2 g
Sodium: 0 mg
Fiber: 2 g

NUTRIENT INTAKE:

43% carbs
4% protein
53% fat

NUTRITION FOR THE DAY

Total Calories: 1321 kcal
Total Fat: 46 g
Saturated Fat: 14.5 g
Total Carbohydrate: 154 g
Protein: 89 g
Sodium: 1282 mg
Fiber: 27 g

NUTRIENT INTAKE:

43% carbs
23% protein
34% fat

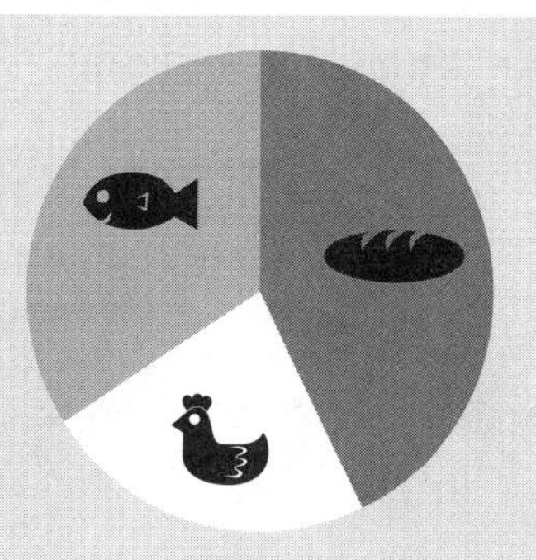

BREAKFAST

► **Berry Blast smoothie (recipe on page 41)**

Total Calories: 188 kcal
Total Fat: 0.5 g
Saturated Fat: 0 g
Total Carbohydrate: 42 g
Protein: 6 g
Sodium: 80 mg
Fiber: 3 g

NUTRIENT INTAKE:

84% carbs
14% protein
2% fat

SNACK 1

► **1 granola bar (Kashi)**

Total Calories: 130 kcal
Total Fat: 5 g
Saturated Fat: 0.5 g
Total Carbohydrate: 20 g
Protein: 5 g
Sodium: 90 mg
Fiber: 4 g

NUTRIENT INTAKE:

55% carbs
14% protein
31% fat

LUNCH

► **Roast Beef and Swiss Wrap**

1 whole wheat tortilla (6 inch)
3 oz low sodium roast beef
1 slice low fat Swiss cheese
2 slices tomato
2 tsp Dijon mustard
½ cup fresh arugula or mixed greens

Total Calories: 338 kcal
Total Fat: 9 g
Saturated Fat: 3 g
Total Carbohydrate: 25 g
Protein: 33 g
Sodium: 546 mg
Fiber: 3 g

NUTRIENT INTAKE:

33% carbs
42% protein
25% fat

SNACK 2

▸ **1 cup chopped pineapple**

Choose a sweet tropical fruit like pineapple to help combat sugary cravings.

Total Calories: 74 kcal
Total Fat: 0 g
Saturated Fat: 0 g
Total Carbohydrate: 20 g
Protein: 1 g
Sodium: 2 mg
Fiber: 2 g

NUTRIENT INTAKE:

95% carbs
4% protein
1% fat

SNACK 3

▸ **6 oz nonfat fruit or vanilla yogurt**

Total Calories: 130 kcal
Total Fat: 0 g
Saturated Fat: 0 g
Total Carbohydrate: 26 g
Protein: 6 g
Sodium: 105 mg
Fiber: 2 g

NUTRIENT INTAKE:

81% carbs
19% protein
0% fat

DINNER

▸ Salmon Caesar Salad

SERVES: 1

4 oz wild salmon, skin removed
1 tsp olive oil
Salt and black pepper

For the dressing:
1 Tbsp olive oil
1 Tbsp lemon juice
½ tsp Dijon mustard
Dash of Worcestershire sauce
1 Tbsp finely grated Parmesan cheese
¼ tsp minced garlic
1 tsp mayonnaise
¼ tsp anchovy paste

2 cups romaine lettuce, chopped
5 cherry tomatoes, halved
Lemon wedges

continued

1. Drizzle salmon with olive oil and season with salt and pepper and roast on a sheet pan in a 400°F oven or wrap in aluminum foil and cook on the grill for 15 minutes until cooked through.
2. In a large bowl combine olive oil, lemon juice, mustard, Worcestershire sauce, Parmesan cheese, garlic, mayonnaise, and anchovy paste—whisk well.
3. Add lettuce and tomato to dressing and toss to coat.
4. Top salad with cooked salmon and serve with lemon wedges.

Total Calories: 378 kcal
Total Fat: 26 g
Saturated Fat: 5 g
Total Carbohydrate: 8 g
Protein: 29 g
Sodium: 331 mg
Fiber: 4 g

NUTRIENT INTAKE:

9% carbs
30% protein
61% fat

SNACK 4 (OPTIONAL)

▸ **1 medium orange**

Total Calories: 62 kcal
Total Fat: 0 g
Saturated Fat: 0 g
Total Carbohydrate: 15 g
Protein: 1 g
Sodium: 0 mg
Fiber: 3 g

NUTRIENT INTAKE:

91% carbs
7% protein
2% fat

NUTRITION FOR THE DAY

Total Calories: 1302 kcal
Total Fat: 41.5 g
Saturated Fat: 9 g
Total Carbohydrate: 157 g
Protein: 82 g
Sodium: 1149 mg
Fiber: 21 g

NUTRIENT INTAKE:

64% carbs
19% protein
17% fat

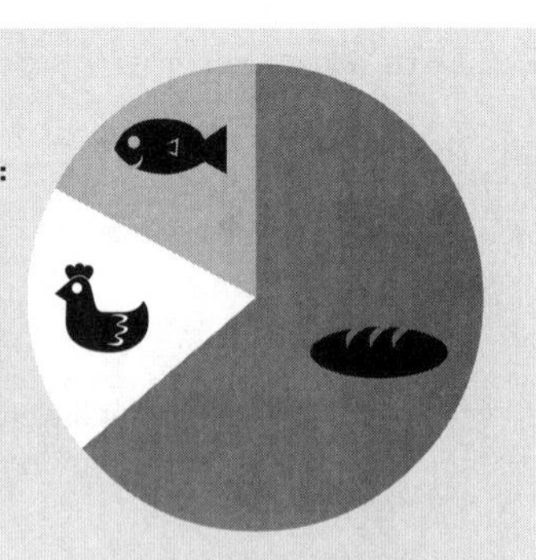

BREAKFAST

- **2 eggs scrambled with ½ cup chopped tomato and 1 Tbsp chopped onion**
- **1 slice whole wheat bread, toasted**

Total Calories: 275 kcal
Total Fat: 11.5 g
Saturated Fat: 3.5 g
Total Carbohydrate: 25 g
Protein: 17 g
Sodium: 294 mg
Fiber: 4 g

NUTRIENT INTAKE:

37% carbs
25% protein
38% fat

SNACK 1

- **6 oz nonfat fruit or vanilla yogurt**

Total Calories: 130 kcal
Total Fat: 0 g
Saturated Fat: 0 g
Total Carbohydrate: 26 g
Protein: 6 g
Sodium: 105 mg
Fiber: 2 g

NUTRIENT INTAKE:

81% carbs
19% protein
0% fat

LUNCH

- **Salad with Tuna**

3 oz canned tuna, in water
1 cup grape tomatoes, halved
½ cup frozen green peas, thawed
2 cups mixed greens
2 Tbsp light vinaigrette salad dressing

Total Calories: 237 kcal
Total Fat: 6 g
Saturated Fat: 0.5 g
Total Carbohydrate: 22 g
Protein: 26 g
Sodium: 960 mg
Fiber: 7 g

NUTRIENT INTAKE:

35% carbs
43% protein
22% fat

SNACK 2

- **3 Tbsp cashews**
- **1 Tbsp raisins**

Total Calories: 175 kcal
Total Fat: 12 g
Saturated Fat: 2 g
Total Carbohydrate: 16 g
Protein: 4 g
Sodium: 5 mg
Fiber: 1 g

NUTRIENT INTAKE:

33% carbs
9% protein
58% fat

SNACK 3

- **1 medium peach**

Total Calories: 38 kcal
Total Fat: 0 g
Saturated Fat: 0 g
Total Carbohydrate: 9 g
Protein: 1 g
Sodium: 0 mg
Fiber: 1.5 g

NUTRIENT INTAKE:

89% carbs
8% protein
5% fat

DINNER

- **4 oz grilled turkey breast**
- **1 sweet potato, diced and roasted with 1 tsp olive oil, salt and pepper**
- **1 cup steamed broccoli**

Sweet potatoes are loaded with beta-carotene and fiber. Baked or roasted, they make a satisfying, guilt-free side dish.

Total Calories: 359 kcal
Total Fat: 6 g
Saturated Fat: 1 g
Total Carbohydrate: 35 g
Protein: 41 g
Sodium: 174 mg
Fiber: 9 g

NUTRIENT INTAKE:

39% carbs
46% protein
15% fat

SNACK 4 (OPTIONAL)

- 2 brown rice cakes

Total Calories: 70 kcal
Total Fat: 0.5 g
Saturated Fat: 0 g
Total Carbohydrate: 15 g
Protein: 1 g
Sodium: 59 mg
Fiber: 1 g

NUTRIENT INTAKE:

NUTRITION FOR THE DAY

Total Calories: 1284 kcal
Total Fat: 36 g
Saturated Fat: 7.5 g
Total Carbohydrate: 147 g
Protein: 97 g
Sodium: 1596 mg
Fiber: 26 g

NUTRIENT INTAKE:

57% carbs

22% protein

21% fat

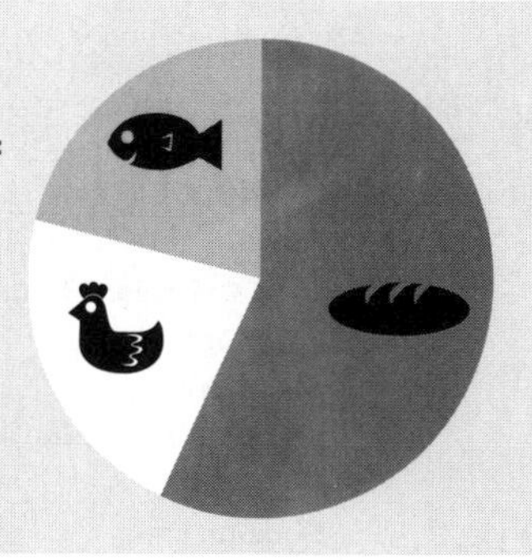

BREAKFAST

- **1 cup whole grain cereal (suggestions: Bran Flakes, Nature's Path Heirloom Flakes)**
- **¾ cup skim milk**
- **½ cup blueberries**

Total Calories: 257 kcal
Total Fat: 2.5 g
Saturated Fat: 0.5 g
Total Carbohydrate: 53 g
Protein: 12 g
Sodium: 79 mg
Fiber: 8 g

NUTRIENT INTAKE:

SNACK 1

- **1 medium peach**

Total Calories: 38 kcal
Total Fat: 0 g
Saturated Fat: 0 g
Total Carbohydrate: 9 g
Protein: 1 g
Sodium: 0 mg
Fiber: 1 g

NUTRIENT INTAKE:

87% carbs
8% protein
5% fat

LUNCH

- **Green Salad with Grilled Chicken**

2 cups mixed greens
½ cup sliced cucumber
¼ cup sliced red onion
½ cup sliced carrots
4 oz grilled chicken breast, sliced
1 Tbsp balsamic vinegar
2 tsp extra-virgin olive oil

Total Calories: 342 kcal
Total Fat: 13 g
Saturated Fat: 2.5 g
Total Carbohydrate: 17 g
Protein: 38 g
Sodium: 162 mg
Fiber: 5 g

NUTRIENT INTAKE:

20% carbs
45% protein
35% fat

SNACK 2

▸ **2 Tbsp cashews**

Total Calories: 98 kcal
Total Fat: 8 g
Saturated Fat: 1.5 g
Total Carbohydrate: 6 g
Protein: 3 g
Sodium: 3 mg
Fiber: 1 g

NUTRIENT INTAKE:

SNACK 3

▸ **1 hard-boiled egg**

Total Calories: 78 kcal
Total Fat: 5 g
Saturated Fat: 1.5 g
Total Carbohydrate: 1 g
Protein: 6 g
Sodium: 62 mg
Fiber: 0 g

NUTRIENT INTAKE:

3% carbs
35% protein
62% fat

DINNER

▸ **Peanut butter noodles with tofu**

***QUICK OPTION MEAL* for peanut butter noodles with tofu** < < < < < < <

6 oz extra-firm tofu, roasted with 2 tsp sesame oil, salt and pepper
1 medium baked sweet potato
1 cup steamed broccoli

Total Calories: 400 kcal
Total Fat: 18.5 g
Saturated Fat: 2.5 g
Total Carbohydrate: 39 g
Protein: 23 g
Sodium: 105 mg
Fiber: 9 g

NUTRIENT INTAKE:

37% carbs
23% protein
40% fat

Peanut Butter Noodles With Tofu

SERVES: 4

12 oz extra-firm tofu, cut into small cubes
1 tsp canola oil

8 oz brown rice pasta (spaghetti or fettuccini) (Tinkyada brand recommended)
1 tsp canola oil
2 cups chopped broccoli
1 cup sliced red bell pepper
2 cups shredded cabbage
½ small onion, sliced
½ tsp grated fresh ginger
1 clove minced garlic
1 tsp chili sauce
1 Tbsp reduced-sodium soy sauce
2 Tbsp natural peanut butter

1. Preheat oven to 400°F.
2. Drain tofu on a paper towel for 5 to 10 minutes.
3. Transfer tofu to a baking sheet, drizzle with 1 tsp canola oil, toss and roast for 25 to 30 minutes, tossing once, until golden.
4. Cook pasta according to package directions. While pasta is cooking, heat remaining canola oil in a large skillet or wok.
5. Add broccoli, pepper, cabbage, onion, ginger, and garlic—toss and cook for 4 to 5 minutes.
6. Add chili sauce, soy sauce, peanut butter, and cooked pasta.
7. Toss well as peanut butter melts and creates a smooth sauce (if pasta appears dry, add a few tablespoons of pasta cooking liquid or water).

Total Calories: 413 kcal
Total Fat: 13 g
Saturated Fat: 2.5 g
Total Carbohydrate: 57 g
Protein: 17 g
Sodium: 177 mg
Fiber: 8 g

NUTRIENT INTAKE:

55% carbs
17% protein
28% fat

SNACK 4 (OPTIONAL)

▸ **1 cup sugar-free, fat-free chocolate pudding**

Total Calories: 60 kcal
Total Fat: 1.5 g
Saturated Fat: 1 g
Total Carbohydrate: 14 g
Protein: 2 g
Sodium: 180 mg
Fiber: 1 g

NUTRIENT INTAKE:

72% carbs
11% protein
17% fat

NUTRITION FOR THE DAY

Total Calories: 1287 kcal
Total Fat: 44 g
Saturated Fat: 10 g
Total Carbohydrate: 157 g
Protein: 79 g
Sodium: 663 mg
Fiber: 25 g

NUTRIENT INTAKE:

48% carbs
20% protein
32% fat

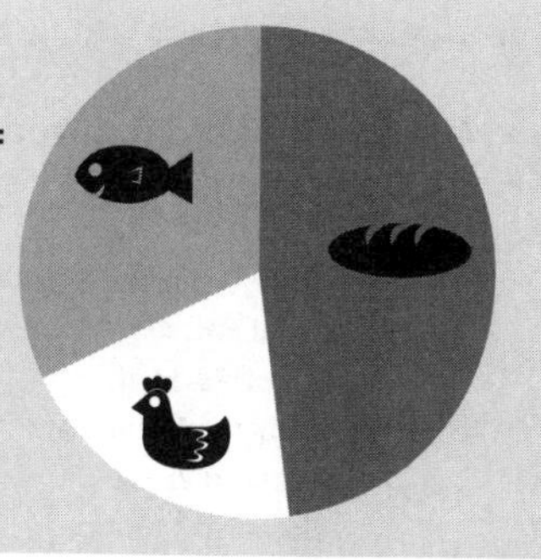

BREAKFAST

- 1 whole wheat English muffin, toasted
- 1 Tbsp almond butter
- 1 medium orange

Total Calories: 297 kcal
Total Fat: 11 g
Saturated Fat: 1 g
Total Carbohydrate: 45 g
Protein: 9 g
Sodium: 492 mg
Fiber: 8 g

NUTRIENT INTAKE:

52% carbs
12% protein
31% fat

SNACK 1

- 4 slices low sodium roast beef, rolled up
- 1 slice low fat Swiss cheese

Total Calories: 140 kcal
Total Fat: 4 g
Saturated Fat: 2 g
Total Carbohydrate: 1 g
Protein: 22 g
Sodium: 113 mg
Fiber: 0 g

NUTRIENT INTAKE:

3% carbs
67% protein
30% fat

LUNCH

- Mediterranean couscous salad

Mediterranean Couscous Salad

SERVES: 1

Prepare a large batch of whole wheat couscous ahead of time for easy assembly of this salad. Just add dry couscous to a pot of boiling water or low sodium broth, cover, and remove from heat. Let it sit for 10 to 15 minutes. One half cup of dry couscous will cook up to about 1¼ cups cooked.

½ cup cooked whole wheat couscous
½ cup cherry tomatoes, halved
½ cup diced cucumber
¼ cup chickpeas, rinsed and drained
1 oz crumbled low fat feta cheese
Fresh parsley
1 tsp honey
2 tsp balsamic vinegar
2 tsp olive oil
⅛ tsp salt
Freshly ground black pepper to taste

1. Combine cooked couscous, tomatoes, cucumber, chickpeas, feta, and parsley—mix to combine.
2. In a small bowl whisk together honey, vinegar, oil, salt and pepper; toss with couscous and serve.

Total Calories: 335 kcal
Total Fat: 14 g
Saturated Fat: 4 g
Total Carbohydrate: 44 g
Protein: 13 g
Sodium: 581 mg
Fiber: 7 g

NUTRIENT INTAKE:

49% carbs

15% protein

36% fat

SNACK 2

▸ **1 cup chopped pineapple**

Total Calories: 74 kcal
Total Fat: 0 g
Saturated Fat: 0 g
Total Carbohydrate: 20 g
Protein: 1 g
Sodium: 2 mg
Fiber: 2 g

NUTRIENT INTAKE:

93% carbs

4% protein

3% fat

SNACK 3

▸ **6 oz nonfat fruit or vanilla yogurt**

Total Calories: 130 kcal
Total Fat: 0 g
Saturated Fat: 0 g
Total Carbohydrate: 26 g
Protein: 6 g
Sodium: 105 mg
Fiber: 2 g

NUTRIENT INTAKE:

81% carbs

19% protein

0% fat

DINNER

- 4 oz grilled pork tenderloin
- 1 cup steamed green beans with 1 tsp olive oil

Lean cuts of pork are a great protein option. Pork is also full of energy-producing B vitamins

Total Calories: 295 kcal
Total Fat: 12 g
Saturated Fat: 3 g
Total Carbohydrate: 10 g
Protein: 37 g
Sodium: 75 mg
Fiber: 4 g

NUTRIENT INTAKE:

13% carbs
50% protein
37% fat

SNACK 4 (OPTIONAL)

- 1 medium peach

Total Calories: 38 kcal
Total Fat: 0 g
Saturated Fat: 0 g
Total Carbohydrate: 9 g
Protein: 1 g
Sodium: 0 mg
Fiber: 1.5 g

NUTRIENT INTAKE:

87% carbs
8% protein
5% fat

NUTRITION FOR THE DAY

Total Calories: 1310 kcal
Total Fat: 42 g
Saturated Fat: 11 g
Total Carbohydrate: 155 g
Protein: 89 g
Sodium: 1368 mg
Fiber: 25 g

NUTRIENT INTAKE:

55% carbs
25% protein
20% fat

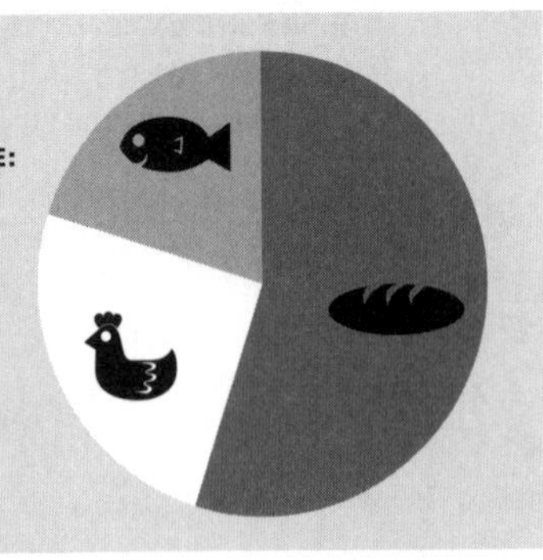

BREAKFAST

- **6 oz nonfat yogurt topped with 1 cup chopped pineapple**

Total Calories: 204 kcal
Total Fat: 0 g
Saturated Fat: 0 g
Total Carbohydrate: 46 g
Protein: 7 g
Sodium: 107 mg
Fiber: 4 g

NUTRIENT INTAKE:

86% carbs
13% protein
1% fat

SNACK 1

- **1 Tbsp almond butter**
- **10 celery strips**

Total Calories: 107 kcal
Total Fat: 9.5 g
Saturated Fat: 1 g
Total Carbohydrate: 5 g
Protein: 3 g
Sodium: 104 mg
Fiber: 1 g

NUTRIENT INTAKE:

16% carbs
9% protein
75% fat

LUNCH

- **Roast Beef and Swiss Sandwich**

1 whole wheat English muffin, toasted
3 oz low sodium roast beef
1 slice low fat Swiss cheese
2 slices tomato
2 tsp Dijon mustard
½ cup fresh arugula or mixed greens

Total Calories: 334 kcal
Total Fat: 7.5 g
Saturated Fat: 3.5 g
Total Carbohydrate: 31 g
Protein: 35 g
Sodium: 678 mg
Fiber: 5 g

NUTRIENT INTAKE:

37% carbs
43% protein
20% fat

SNACK 2

▸ **1 medium orange**

Total Calories: 62 kcal
Total Fat: 0 g
Saturated Fat: 0 g
Total Carbohydrate: 15 g
Protein: 1 g
Sodium: 0 mg
Fiber: 3 g

NUTRIENT INTAKE:

90% carbs
8% protein
2% fat

SNACK 3

▸ **1 hard-boiled egg**

Total Calories: 78 kcal
Total Fat: 5.5 g
Saturated Fat: 1.5 g
Total Carbohydrate: 1 g
Protein: 6 g
Sodium: 62 mg
Fiber: 0 g

NUTRIENT INTAKE:

3% carbs
35% protein
62% fat

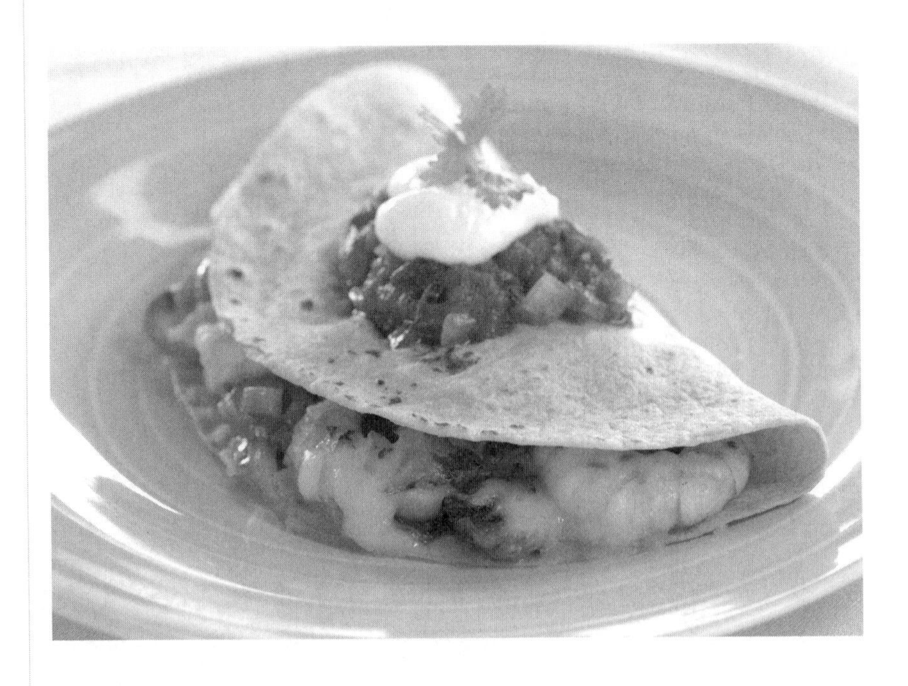

DINNER

▸ Shrimp Quesadilla

SERVES: 1

1 tsp canola oil
1 clove chopped garlic
3 oz raw shrimp, peeled and deveined
¼ cup thinly sliced red onion
¼ cup diced bell pepper
¼ cup sliced mushrooms
1 cup baby spinach
¼ tsp Worcestershire sauce
¼ cup low fat shredded cheese
1 whole wheat tortilla
Nonstick cooking spray

2 Tbsp salsa
2 Tbsp nonfat Greek yogurt

1. Heat oil in a nonstick skillet over medium heat.
2. Add garlic and shrimp and cook for 2 minutes.
3. Add onion, pepper, mushrooms, spinach, and Worcestershire sauce; cook for an additional 5 minutes; transfer to a bowl.
4. Spray the same skillet with nonstick cooking spray, place tortilla in pan, and top half with shrimp mixture and cheese.
5. Fold tortilla in half and cook for 2 minutes per side, pressing down with a spatula until tortilla is golden and cheese is melted.
6. Serve topped with salsa and yogurt.

Total Calories: 396 kcal
Total Fat: 11 g
Saturated Fat: 2 g
Total Carbohydrate: 37 g
Protein: 32 g
Sodium: 741 mg
Fiber: 6 g

NUTRIENT INTAKE:

38% carbs
35% protein
27% fat

SNACK 4 (OPTIONAL)

- **2 Tbsp cashews**

Total Calories: 99 kcal
Total Fat: 8 g
Saturated Fat: 1.5 g
Total Carbohydrate: 6 g
Protein: 3 g
Sodium: 3 mg
Fiber: 1 g

NUTRIENT INTAKE:

21% carbs
11% protein
68% fat

NUTRITION FOR THE DAY

Total Calories: 1276 kcal
Total Fat: 42 g
Saturated Fat: 9.5 g
Total Carbohydrate: 139 g
Protein: 89 g
Sodium: 1693 mg
Fiber: 20 g

NUTRIENT INTAKE:

42% carbs
22% protein
36% fat

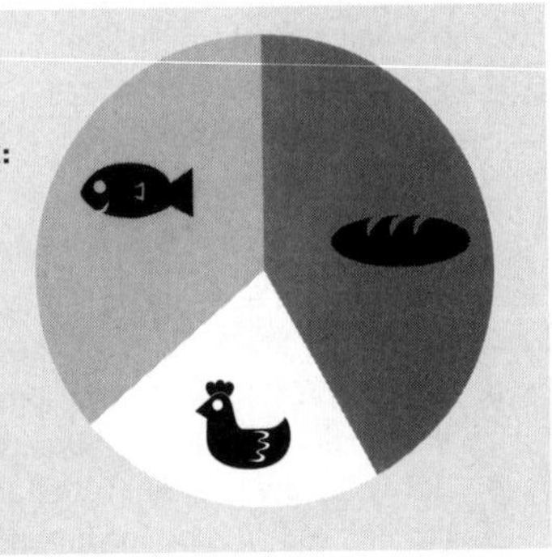

BREAKFAST

▸ Egg and Cheese

1 egg, cooked any style
1 slice low fat Swiss cheese
1 slice tomato

Total Calories: 261 kcal
Total Fat: 8 g
Saturated Fat: 3 g
Total Carbohydrate: 29 g
Protein: 20 g
Sodium: 564 mg
Fiber: 5 g

NUTRIENT INTAKE:

43% carbs
31% protein
26% fat

SNACK 1

▸ 2 Tbsp cashews
▸ 1 Tbsp raisins

Total Calories: 126 kcal
Total Fat: 8 g
Saturated Fat: 1.5 g
Total Carbohydrate: 13 g
Protein: 3 g
Sodium: 4 mg
Fiber: 1 g

NUTRIENT INTAKE:

38% carbs
9% protein
53% fat

LUNCH

▸ Chicken Salad with Chickpeas

2 cups chopped lettuce
3 oz grilled chicken breast, cubed
½ cup sliced cucumber
¼ cup chickpeas
2 Tbsp light vinaigrette dressing

Total Calories: 275 kcal
Total Fat: 8 g
Saturated Fat: 1.5 g
Total Carbohydrate: 19 g
Protein: 31 g
Sodium: 734 mg
Fiber: 4 g

NUTRIENT INTAKE:

29% carbs
45% protein
26% fat

SNACK 2

- 6 oz nonfat fruit or vanilla yogurt

Total Calories: 130 kcal
Total Fat: 0 g
Saturated Fat: 0 g
Total Carbohydrate: 26 g
Protein: 6 g
Sodium: 105 mg
Fiber: 2 g

NUTRIENT INTAKE:

81% carbs
19% protein
0% fat

SNACK 3

- 1 granola bar (Kashi)

Total Calories: 130 kcal
Total Fat: 5 g
Saturated Fat: 0.5 g
Total Carbohydrate: 20 g
Protein: 5 g
Sodium: 90 mg
Fiber: 4 g

NUTRIENT INTAKE:

55% carbs
14% protein
31% fat

DINNER

- 4 oz cooked chicken sausage
- 1 cup steamed broccoli
- ½ cup cooked whole wheat couscous

Chicken sausage is much lower in fat than traditional pork sausages, and you can find them in a variety of flavors.

Total Calories: 329 kcal
Total Fat: 11 g
Saturated Fat: 3.5 g
Total Carbohydrate: 37 g
Protein: 26 g
Sodium: 724 mg
Fiber: 9 g

NUTRIENT INTAKE:

44% carbs
30% protein
26% fat

SNACK 4 (OPTIONAL)

- **1 cup sugar-free, fat-free chocolate pudding**

Total Calories: 60 kcal
Total Fat: 1.5 g
Saturated Fat: 1 g
Total Carbohydrate: 14 g
Protein: 2 g
Sodium: 180 mg
Fiber: 1 g

NUTRIENT INTAKE:

72% carbs
11% protein
17% fat

NUTRITION FOR THE DAY

Total Calories: 1311 kcal
Total Fat: 41.5 g
Saturated Fat: 11 g
Total Carbohydrate: 158 g
Protein: 93 g
Sodium: 2300 mg
Fiber: 25 g

NUTRIENT INTAKE:

51% carbs
23% protein
26% fat

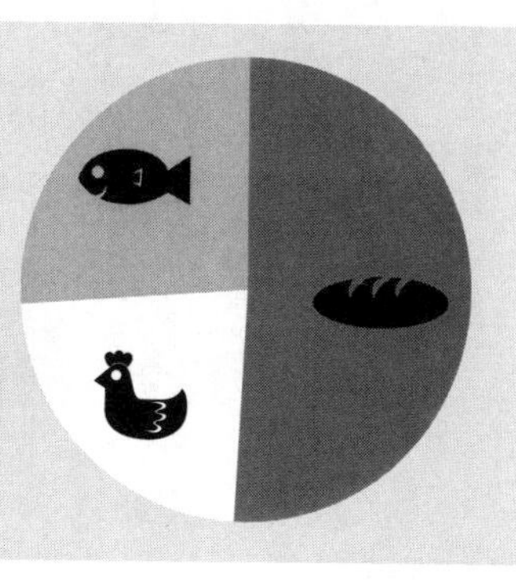

BREAKFAST

- ¾ cup skim milk
- Buttermilk blueberry pancakes

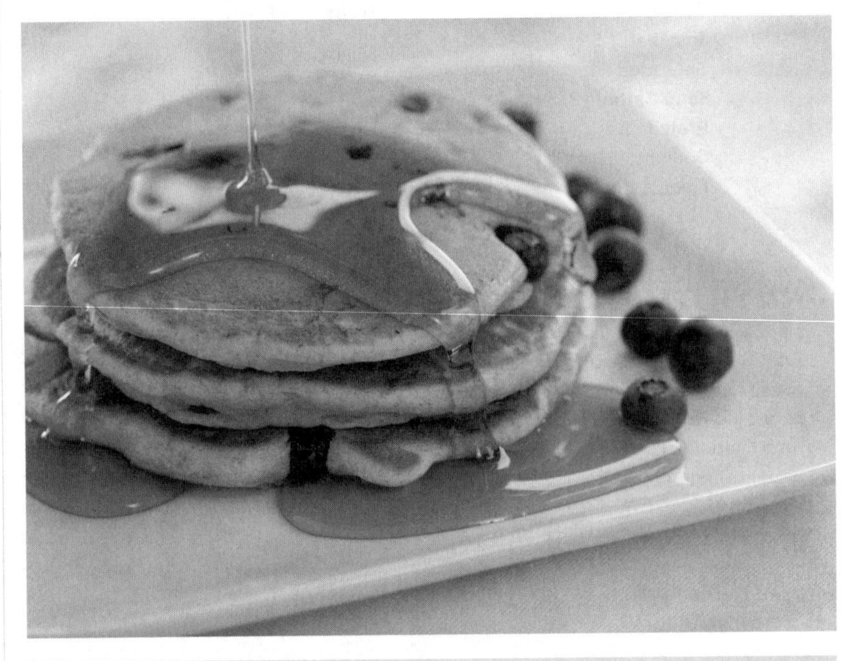

Buttermilk Blueberry Pancakes

SERVES: 4 (3 PANCAKES AND 2 TBSP PURE MAPLE SYRUP PER SERVING)

½ cup whole wheat flour
½ cup all-purpose flour
1 Tbsp sugar
1 tsp baking powder
½ tsp baking soda
Pinch salt
1 egg, lightly beaten
1 cup low fat buttermilk
¼ cup water
1 tsp vanilla extract
2 tsp canola oil
¾ cup blueberries
Nonstick cooking spray
8 Tbsp pure maple syrup

Buttermilk is a perfect low fat replacement for some of the fat in pancakes and baked goods.

1. In a large bowl, sift together flours, sugar, baking powder, baking soda, and salt.
2. Add egg, buttermilk, water, vanilla, and oil; mix until just combined. Fold in blueberries, set aside.
3. Heat a nonstick pan or griddle over medium heat, spray with nonstick spray.
4. Pour ¼ cup of batter for each pancake into pan and cook for 2 minutes per side until golden.
5. Serve topped with maple syrup.

Total Calories: 372 kcal
Total Fat: 5 g
Saturated Fat: 1 g
Total Carbohydrate: 69 g
Protein: 13 g
Sodium: 477 mg
Fiber: 3 g

NUTRIENT INTAKE:

74% carbs
14% protein
12% fat

SNACK 1

- **1 medium peach**

Total Calories: 38 kcal
Total Fat: 0 g
Saturated Fat: 0 g
Total Carbohydrate: 9 g
Protein: 1 g
Sodium: 0 mg
Fiber: 1.5 g

NUTRIENT INTAKE:

87% carbs
8% protein
5% fat

LUNCH

- **1 medium baked sweet potato topped with ½ cup steamed broccoli and 1 Tbsp nonfat Greek yogurt**
- **1½ cups mixed greens with 1 Tbsp low fat vinaigrette**

Total Calories: 174 kcal
Total Fat: 2.5 g
Saturated Fat: 0 g
Total Carbohydrate: 34 g
Protein: 6 g
Sodium: 336 mg
Fiber: 8 g

NUTRIENT INTAKE:

74% carbs
14% protein
12% fat

SNACK 2

- 1 brown rice cake
- 1 Tbsp almond butter

Total Calories: 136 kcal
Total Fat: 10 g
Saturated Fat: 1 g
Total Carbohydrate: 11 g
Protein: 3 g
Sodium: 101 mg
Fiber: 1 g

NUTRIENT INTAKE:

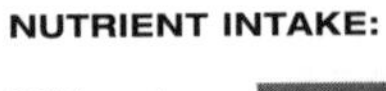

30% carbs
9% protein
61% fat

SNACK 3

- 2 oz low sodium roast beef, rolled up
- 1 slice low fat Swiss cheese

Total Calories: 140 kcal
Total Fat: 4 g
Saturated Fat: 2 g
Total Carbohydrate: 1 g
Protein: 22 g
Sodium: 113 mg
Fiber: 0 g

NUTRIENT INTAKE:

3% carbs
67% protein
30% fat

DINNER

- 4 oz grilled chicken breast
- 1 cup steamed green beans with 1 tsp olive oil and 1 tsp lemon juice

Total Calories: 271 kcal
Total Fat: 9 g
Saturated Fat: 2 g
Total Carbohydrate: 10 g
Protein: 38 g
Sodium: 85 mg
Fiber: 4 g

NUTRIENT INTAKE:

15% carbs
56% protein
29% fat

SNACK 4 (OPTIONAL)

▸ **2 Tbsp cashews**

Total Calories: 98 kcal
Total Fat: 8 g
Saturated Fat: 1.5 g
Total Carbohydrate: 6 g
Protein: 3 g
Sodium: 3 mg
Fiber: 1 g

NUTRIENT INTAKE:

21% carbs
11% protein
68% fat

NUTRITION FOR THE DAY

Total Calories: 1232 kcal
Total Fat: 39 g
Saturated Fat: 8 g
Total Carbohydrate: 140 g
Protein: 86 g
Sodium: 1113 mg
Fiber: 18 g

NUTRIENT INTAKE:

43% carbs
26% protein
31% fat

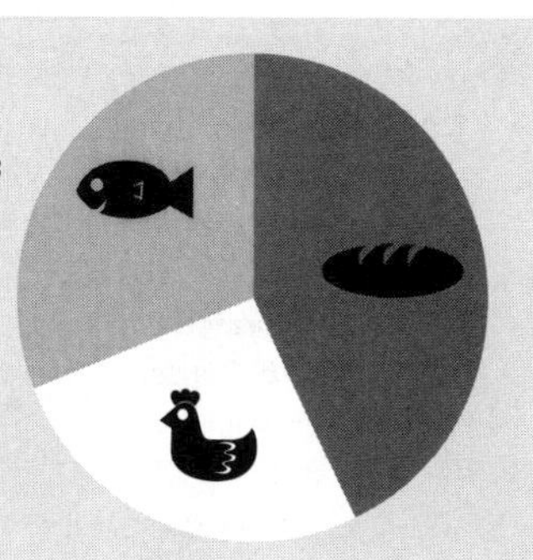

BREAKFAST

- **1 cup cooked steel-cut oatmeal topped with ½ cup sliced strawberries, 2 Tbsp chopped almonds, and 2 tsp maple syrup**

Total Calories: 283 kcal
Total Fat: 9 g
Saturated Fat: 1 g
Total Carbohydrate: 46 g
Protein: 8 g
Sodium: 2 mg
Fiber: 9 g

NUTRIENT INTAKE:

62% carbs
11% protein
27% fat

SNACK 1

- **1 hard-boiled egg**

Total Calories: 78 kcal
Total Fat: 5 g
Saturated Fat: 1.5 g
Total Carbohydrate: 1 g
Protein: 6 g
Sodium: 62 mg
Fiber: 0 g

NUTRIENT INTAKE:

3% carbs
33% protein
64% fat

LUNCH

- **Chicken and Rice Bowl**

4 oz grilled chicken breast
3 Tbsp diced avocado
2 Tbsp salsa
½ cup cooked brown rice

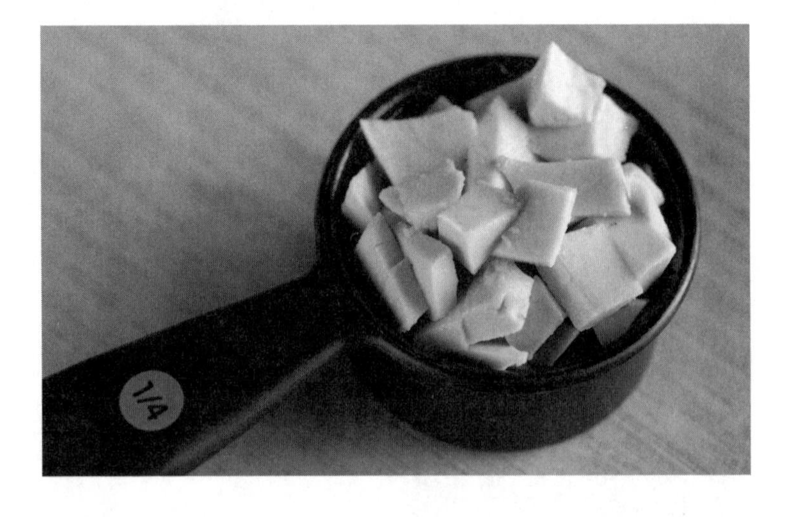

Total Calories: 349 kcal
Total Fat: 9 g
Saturated Fat: 2 g
Total Carbohydrate: 27 g
Protein: 39 g
Sodium: 289 mg
Fiber: 4 g

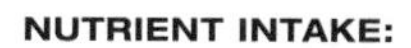

NUTRIENT INTAKE:

31% carbs
45% protein
24% fat

SNACK 2

- **1 medium pear**
- **10 almonds**

Total Calories: 166 kcal
Total Fat: 6 g
Saturated Fat: 0.5 g
Total Carbohydrate: 28 g
Protein: 3 g
Sodium: 2 mg
Fiber: 7 g

NUTRIENT INTAKE:

62% carbs
7% protein
31% fat

SNACK 3

- **1 part-skim mozzarella string cheese**

Total Calories: 80 kcal
Total Fat: 6 g
Saturated Fat: 3.5 g
Total Carbohydrate: 1 g
Protein: 7 g
Sodium: 220 mg
Fiber: 0 g

NUTRIENT INTAKE:

5% carbs
33% protein
62% fat

DINNER

- **4 oz grilled chicken sausage**
- **Sautéed zucchini**

Sautéed Zucchini

SERVES: 1

1 tsp olive oil
1 medium zucchini
½ tsp minced garlic
¼ cup thinly sliced onion
¼ tsp dried oregano or 1 tsp fresh oregano
Pinch red pepper flakes
⅛ tsp salt

continued

Heat oil in a skillet over medium heat, add remaining ingredients, and sauté for 10 minutes until zucchini is tender. If mixture appears dry, add a splash of water or broth.

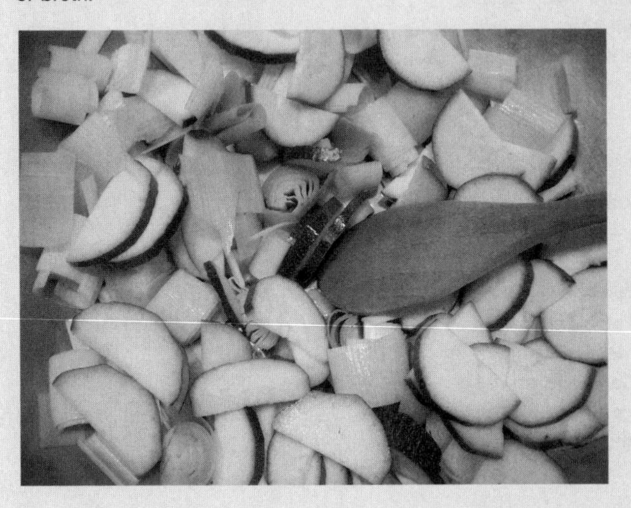

Total Calories: 191 kcal
Total Fat: 11 g
Saturated Fat: 3 g
Total Carbohydrate: 13 g
Protein: 14 g
Sodium: 551 mg
Fiber: 3 g

NUTRIENT INTAKE:

26% carbs
27% protein
47% fat

DESSERT

▸ Peach Frozen Yogurt

MAKES 8 HALF-CUP SERVINGS

If peaches aren't in season, use frozen, unsweetened peaches that have been thawed. This recipe works for almost any kind of fresh fruit.

5 medium ripe peaches, peeled and diced (about 3 cups), divided
1 cup plain low fat yogurt
1 cup plain low fat Greek yogurt
½ cup sugar

1. To peel peaches, cut a small, shallow "x" mark onto the bottom of each peach.
2. Drop peaches into a pot of boiling water for 30 seconds.
3. Remove and place directly into a bowl of ice water (this will loosen the skin).
4. Peel skin away, remove pit, and dice.
5. Place 2 cups diced peaches, yogurts, and sugar in a food processor and pulse until combined.

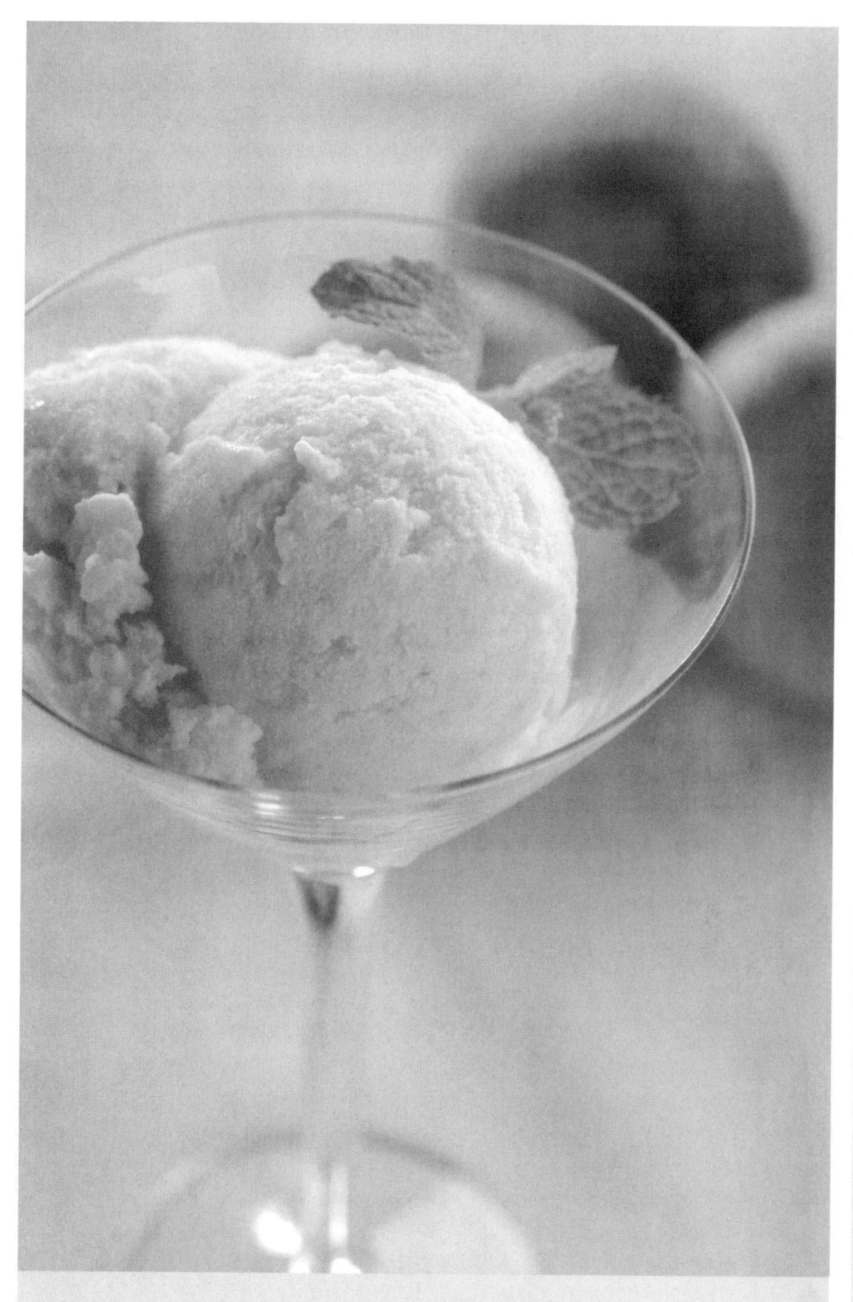

6. Transfer mixture to an ice cream maker and process according to the manufacturer's suggestions. If you don't have an ice cream maker, freeze the mixture for 1 to 2 hours and then process again in the food processor before serving.

Total Calories: 110 kcal
Total Fat: 1 g
Saturated Fat: 0.5 g
Total Carbohydrate: 22 g
Protein: 4 g
Sodium: 33 mg
Fiber: 1 g

NUTRIENT INTAKE:

76% carbs
15% protein
9% fat

NUTRITION FOR THE DAY

Total Calories: 1256 kcal
Total Fat: 47 g
Saturated Fat: 12 g
Total Carbohydrate: 137 g
Protein: 82 g
Sodium: 1159 mg
Fiber: 24 g

NUTRIENT INTAKE:

38% carbs
24% protein
38% fat

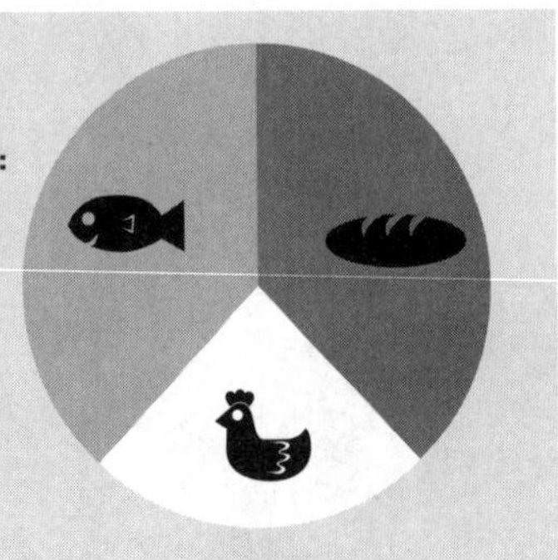

BREAKFAST

- 1 slice whole wheat bread, toasted
- 1 Tbsp natural peanut butter
- 1 medium banana

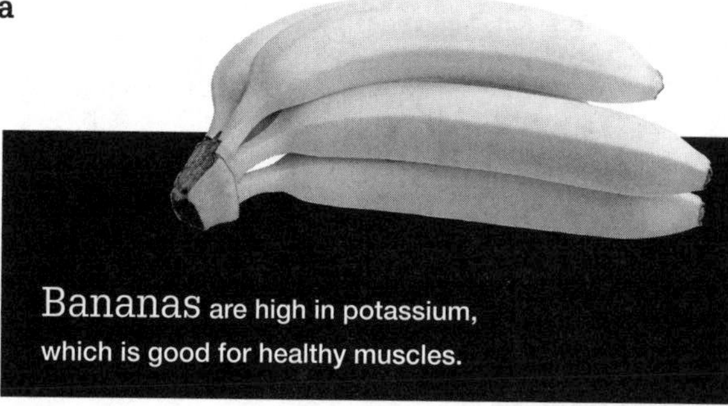

Total Calories: 320 kcal
Total Fat: 10 g
Saturated Fat: 2 g
Total Carbohydrate: 50 g
Protein: 9 g
Sodium: 166 mg
Fiber: 8 g

NUTRIENT INTAKE:

61% carbs
11% protein
28% fat

SNACK 1

- 1 medium grapefruit

Total Calories: 82 kcal
Total Fat: 0 g
Saturated Fat: 0 g
Total Carbohydrate: 21 g
Protein: 2 g
Sodium: 0 mg
Fiber: 3 g

NUTRIENT INTAKE:

90% carbs
7% protein
3% fat

LUNCH

- 1½ cups low sodium lentil or black bean soup (Amy's)
- 2 cups mixed greens topped with 2 tsp olive oil and 2 tsp balsamic vinegar

Total Calories: 371 kcal
Total Fat: 19.5 g
Saturated Fat: 2.5 g
Total Carbohydrate: 40 g
Protein: 12 g
Sodium: 537 mg
Fiber: 12 g

NUTRIENT INTAKE:

42% carbs
12% protein
46% fat

SNACK 2

- 2 oz low sodium turkey breast, rolled up

Total Calories: 60 kcal
Total Fat: 1 g
Saturated Fat: 0 g
Total Carbohydrate: 0 g
Protein: 13 g
Sodium: 350 mg
Fiber: 0 g

NUTRIENT INTAKE:

0% carbs
91% protein
9% fat

SNACK 3

- 10 baby carrots
- ¼ cup hummus

Hummus is a great combo of fiber, protein, and healthy carbs and a great hunger-fighting snack.

Total Calories: 128 kcal
Total Fat: 5.5 g
Saturated Fat: 1 g
Total Carbohydrate: 16 g
Protein: 5 g
Sodium: 290 mg
Fiber: 5 g

NUTRIENT INTAKE:

48% carbs
15% protein
37% fat

DINNER

- 5 oz grilled chicken breast
- ½ cup cooked brown rice
- 1 cup steamed broccoli with lemon juice

Total Calories: 397 kcal
Total Fat: 6.5 g
Saturated Fat: 2 g
Total Carbohydrate: 34 g
Protein: 50 g
Sodium: 174 mg
Fiber: 7 g

NUTRIENT INTAKE:

34% carbs
51% protein
15% fat

SNACK 4 (OPTIONAL)

▸ **1 cup air-popped popcorn**

Total Calories: 31 kcal
Total Fat: 0 g
Saturated Fat: 0 g
Total Carbohydrate: 6 g
Protein: 1 g
Sodium: 1 mg
Fiber: 1 g

NUTRIENT INTAKE:

77% carbs

13% protein

10% fat

NUTRITION FOR THE DAY

Total Calories: 1386 kcal
Total Fat: 43 g
Saturated Fat: 7 g
Total Carbohydrate: 167 g
Protein: 91 g
Sodium: 1511 mg
Fiber: 35 g

NUTRIENT INTAKE:

50% carbs

29% protein

21% fat

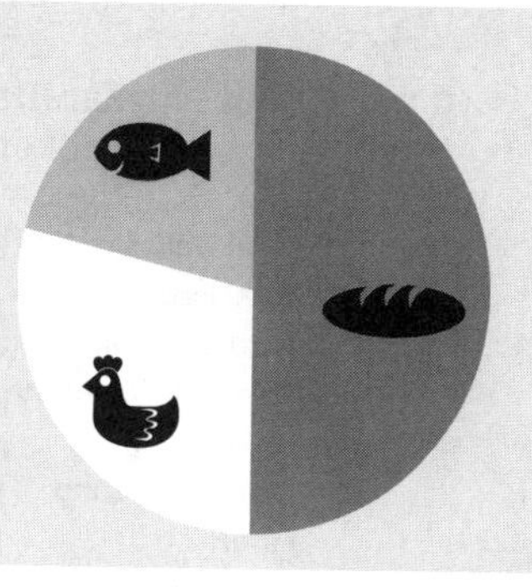

BREAKFAST

- **1 cup nonfat Greek yogurt topped with ½ cup raspberries and ½ cup whole grain cereal**

Total Calories: 229 kcal
Total Fat: 1 g
Saturated Fat: 0 g
Total Carbohydrate: 33 g
Protein: 24 g
Sodium: 86 mg
Fiber: 7 g

NUTRIENT INTAKE:

55% carbs
40% protein
5% fat

SNACK 1

- **1 part-skim mozzarella string cheese**
- **5 whole wheat crackers**

Total Calories: 130 kcal
Total Fat: 7 g
Saturated Fat: 3.5 g
Total Carbohydrate: 9 g
Protein: 9 g
Sodium: 337 mg
Fiber: 2 g

NUTRIENT INTAKE:

27% carbs
25% protein
48% fat

LUNCH

- **Guacamole Salad with Chicken**

2 cups chopped lettuce
½ cup chopped bell pepper
5 cherry tomatoes, halved
2 Tbsp diced avocado
1 Tbsp fresh cilantro (optional)
4 oz grilled chicken breast, sliced
1 tsp olive oil
Fresh lime juice to taste

Total Calories: 308 kcal
Total Fat: 12 g
Saturated Fat: 2 g
Total Carbohydrate: 13 g
Protein: 39 g
Sodium: 97 mg
Fiber: 5 g

NUTRIENT INTAKE:

15% carbs
50% protein
35% fat

SNACK 2

- 1 medium apple

Total Calories: 72 kcal
Total Fat: 0 g
Saturated Fat: 0 g
Total Carbohydrate: 19 g
Protein: 0 g
Sodium: 1 mg
Fiber: 3 g

NUTRIENT INTAKE:
95% carbs
3% protein
2% fat

SNACK 3

- 10 almonds

Total Calories: 69 kcal
Total Fat: 6 g
Saturated Fat: 0.5 g
Total Carbohydrate: 2 g
Protein: 3 g
Sodium: 0 mg
Fiber: 1 g

NUTRIENT INTAKE:
14% carbs
13% protein
73% fat

DINNER

- Chili-rubbed flank steak with oven fries
- 1 cup sliced cucumber

QUICK OPTION MEAL for chili-rubbed flank steak with oven fries < < < < < < < < < < <

4 oz grilled flank steak
1 cup steamed broccoli
½ cup cooked whole wheat couscous

Calories: 380 kcal
Total Fat: 10.5 g
Saturated Fat: 4 g
Total Carbohydrate: 35 g
Protein: 39 g
Sodium: 127 mg
Fiber: 8 g

Nutrient intake:
35% carbs
40% protein
25% fat

Chili-rubbed Steak with Oven Fries

SERVES: 4

1 lb flank steak

Dry Rub:
1 Tbsp chili powder
1 Tbsp light brown sugar
1 tsp kosher salt
1 tsp black pepper
2 tsp lemon or lime zest

4 Yukon gold potatoes, cut lengthwise into strips
2 tsp olive oil
¼ tsp salt
⅛ tsp black pepper

1. Preheat oven to 400°F.
2. In a small bowl mix together dry rub ingredients.
3. Rub mixture onto both sides of flank steak, wrap up, and refrigerate for at least 20 minutes (or up to 4 hours).

Dry Rub—a combo of dried spices packs tons of flavor and few calories to meats, fish, and veggies.

4. Place potatoes on a baking sheet, drizzle with oil, season with salt and pepper, toss and bake for 35 to 40 minutes, turning once, until golden brown.
5. Grill or broil steak for 7 to 8 minutes per side or until cooked as desired.

Serve with 1 cup sliced cucumber topped with 1 tsp olive oil and lemon juice

Total Calories: 368 kcal
Total Fat: 13 g
Saturated Fat: 3 g
Total Carbohydrate: 35 g
Protein: 29 g
Sodium: 243 mg
Fiber: 5 g

NUTRIENT INTAKE:

38% carbs
31% protein
31% fat

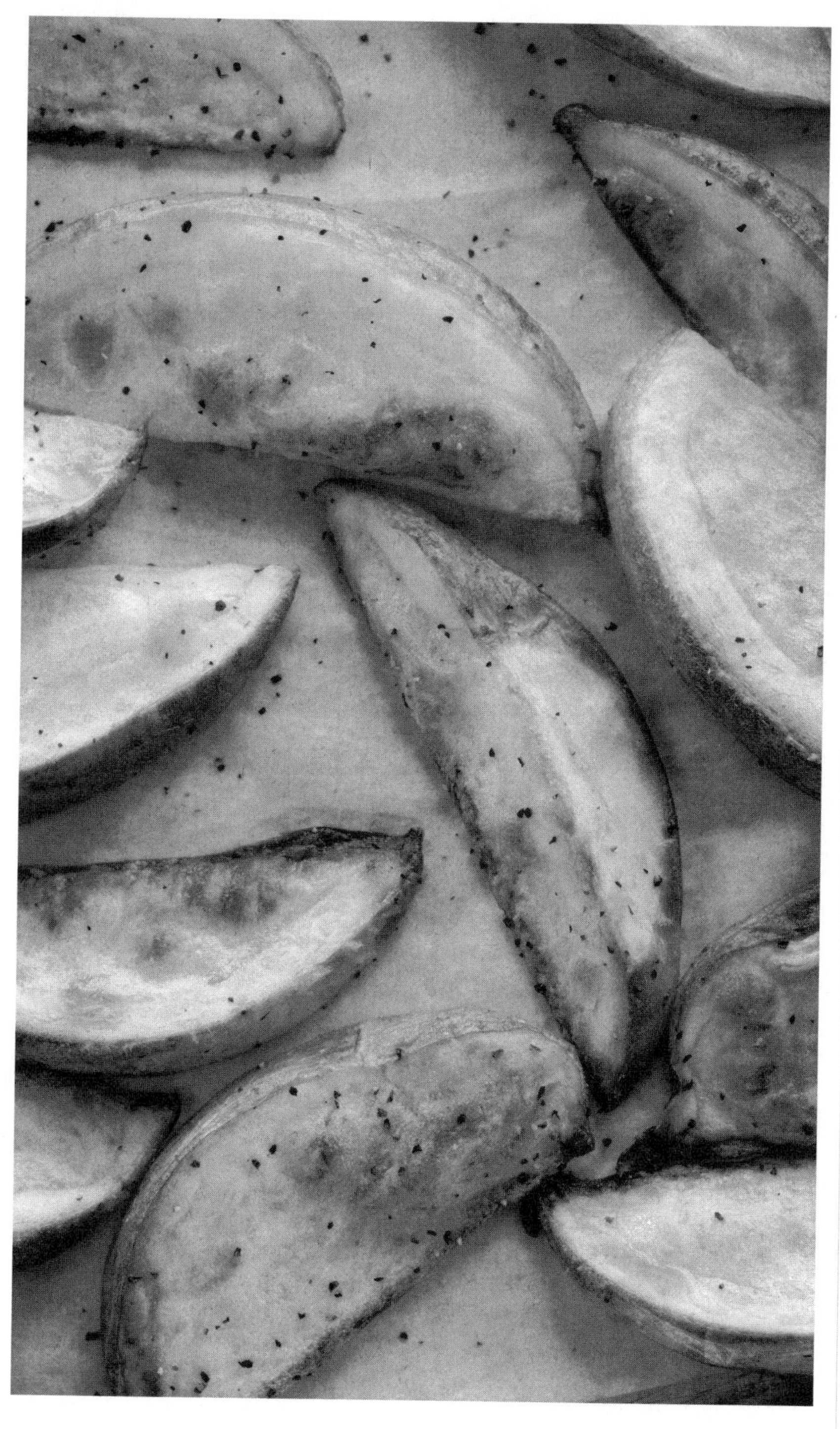

SNACK 4 (OPTIONAL)

► ½ medium grapefruit

Total Calories: 41 kcal
Total Fat: 0 g
Saturated Fat: 0 g
Total Carbohydrate: 10 g
Protein: 1 g
Sodium: 0 mg
Fiber: 1 g

NUTRIENT INTAKE:

90% carbs
7% protein
3% fat

NUTRITION FOR THE DAY

Total Calories: 1211 kcal
Total Fat: 40 g
Saturated Fat: 10 g
Total Carbohydrate: 121 g
Protein: 102 g
Sodium: 779 mg
Fiber: 25 g

NUTRIENT INTAKE:

48% carbs
24% protein
28% fat

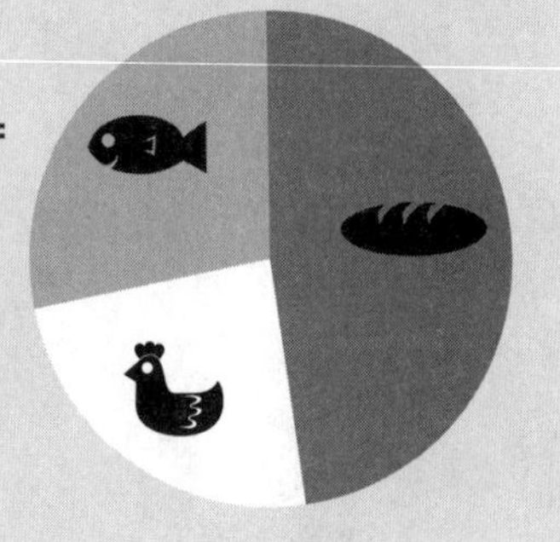

BREAKFAST

- 1 egg + 2 egg whites, scrambled with ½ cup chopped bell pepper and 2 Tbsp grated Parmesan cheese
- 1 cup skim milk

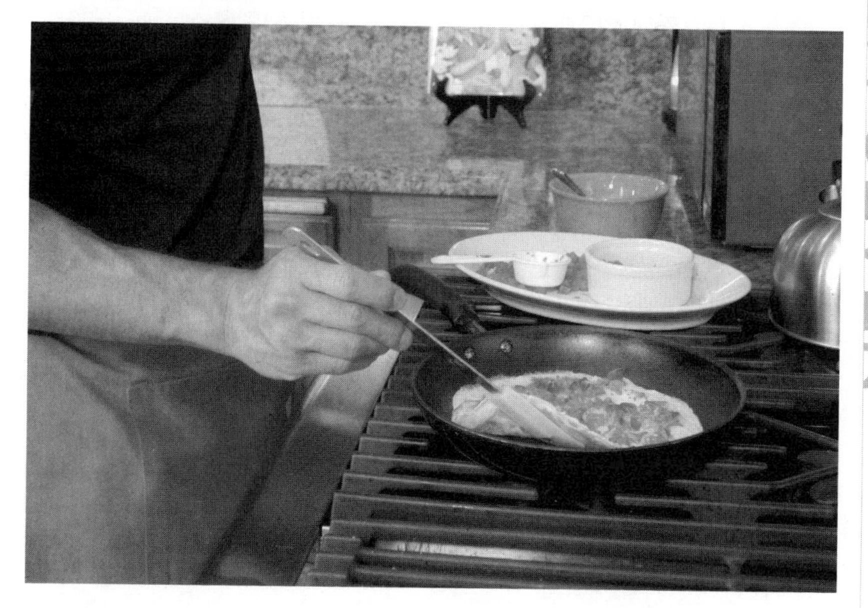

Total Calories: 251 kcal
Total Fat: 8.5 g
Saturated Fat: 3.5 g
Total Carbohydrate: 16 g
Protein: 26 g
Sodium: 463 mg
Fiber: 1 g

NUTRIENT INTAKE:

28% carbs
42% protein
30% fat

SNACK 1

- ½ cup nonfat Greek yogurt
- 1 medium pear, diced

Total Calories: 156 kcal
Total Fat: 0 g
Saturated Fat: 0 g
Total Carbohydrate: 30 g
Protein: 11 g
Sodium: 44 mg
Fiber: 5 g

NUTRIENT INTAKE:

73% carbs
26% protein
1% fat

LUNCH

- Tuna and apples (recipe on page 145)
- 2 cups mixed greens

Total Calories: 309 kcal
Total Fat: 12.5 g
Saturated Fat: 1.5 g
Total Carbohydrate: 17 g
Protein: 34 g
Sodium: 745 mg
Fiber: 3 g

NUTRIENT INTAKE:

22% carbs
42% protein
36% fat

SNACK 2

- 1 medium apple or pear
- 1 Tbsp natural peanut butter

Total Calories: 177 kcal
Total Fat: 9 g
Saturated Fat: 1.5 g
Total Carbohydrate: 22 g
Protein: 4 g
Sodium: 16 mg
Fiber: 5 g

NUTRIENT INTAKE:

48% carbs
9% protein
43% fat

SNACK 3

- 1 cup air-popped popcorn

Total Calories: 31 kcal
Total Fat: 0 g
Saturated Fat: 0 g
Total Carbohydrate: 6 g
Protein: 1 g
Sodium: 1 mg
Fiber: 1 g

NUTRIENT INTAKE:

80% carbs
9% protein
11% fat

DINNER

- Tofu stir-fry (recipe on page 119)
- ½ cup cooked brown rice

Total Calories: 407 kcal
Total Fat: 16.5 g
Saturated Fat: 2 g
Total Carbohydrate: 48 g
Protein: 19 g
Sodium: 561 mg
Fiber: 10 g

NUTRIENT INTAKE:

46% carbs
18% protein
36% fat

SNACK 4 (OPTIONAL)

- ½ frozen banana

Total Calories: 53 kcal
Total Fat: 0 g
Saturated Fat: 0 g
Total Carbohydrate: 13 g
Protein: 1 g
Sodium: 1 mg
Fiber: 2 g

NUTRIENT INTAKE:

93% carbs
4% protein
3% fat

NUTRITION FOR THE DAY

Total Calories: 1390 kcal
Total Fat: 47 g
Saturated Fat: 9 g
Total Carbohydrate: 155 g
Protein: 96 g
Sodium: 1790 mg
Fiber: 27 g

NUTRIENT INTAKE:

56% carbs
21% protein
23% fat

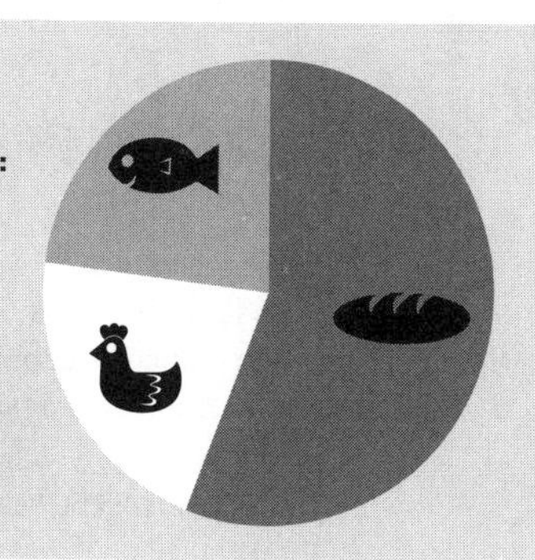

BREAKFAST

1 cup whole grain cereal (suggestions: Bran Flakes, Nature's Path Heirloom Flakes)
¾ cup skim milk
½ cup raspberries

Total Calories: 248 kcal
Total Fat: 2.5 g
Saturated Fat: 0.5 g
Total Carbohydrate: 50 g
Protein: 12 g
Sodium: 79 mg
Fiber: 10 g

NUTRIENT INTAKE:

SNACK 1

- **1 medium pear**
- **2 oz low sodium turkey breast**

Total Calories: 156 kcal
Total Fat: 1 g
Saturated Fat: 0 g
Total Carbohydrate: 26 g
Protein: 14 g
Sodium: 352 mg
Fiber: 5 g

NUTRIENT INTAKE:

62% carbs
32% protein
6% fat

LUNCH

- **Tofu Wrap**

1 whole wheat tortilla
3 oz tofu (from tofu stir-fry, Day 4 dinner)
½ cup chopped lettuce or cabbage
2 Tbsp diced avocado with fresh lime juice to taste

Total Calories: 260 kcal
Total Fat: 10 g
Saturated Fat: 1 g
Total Carbohydrate: 27 g
Protein: 13 g
Sodium: 176 mg
Fiber: 5 g

NUTRIENT INTAKE:

42% carbs
21% protein
37% fat

SNACK 2

- 10 baby carrots
- ¼ cup hummus

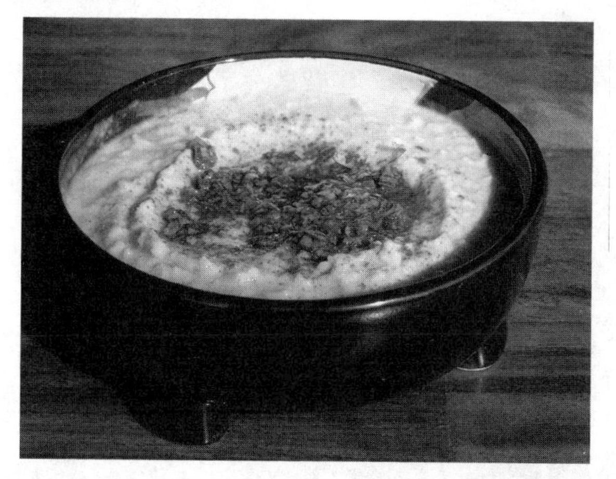

Total Calories: 128 kcal
Total Fat: 5.5 g
Saturated Fat: 1 g
Total Carbohydrate: 16 g
Protein: 5 g
Sodium: 290 mg
Fiber: 5 g

NUTRIENT INTAKE:

47% carbs
15% protein
38% fat

SNACK 3

- 1 part-skim mozzarella string cheese

Total Calories: 80 kcal
Total Fat: 6 g
Saturated Fat: 3.5 g
Total Carbohydrate: 1 g
Protein: 7 g
Sodium: 220 mg
Fiber: 0 g

NUTRIENT INTAKE:

5% carbs
33% protein
63% fat

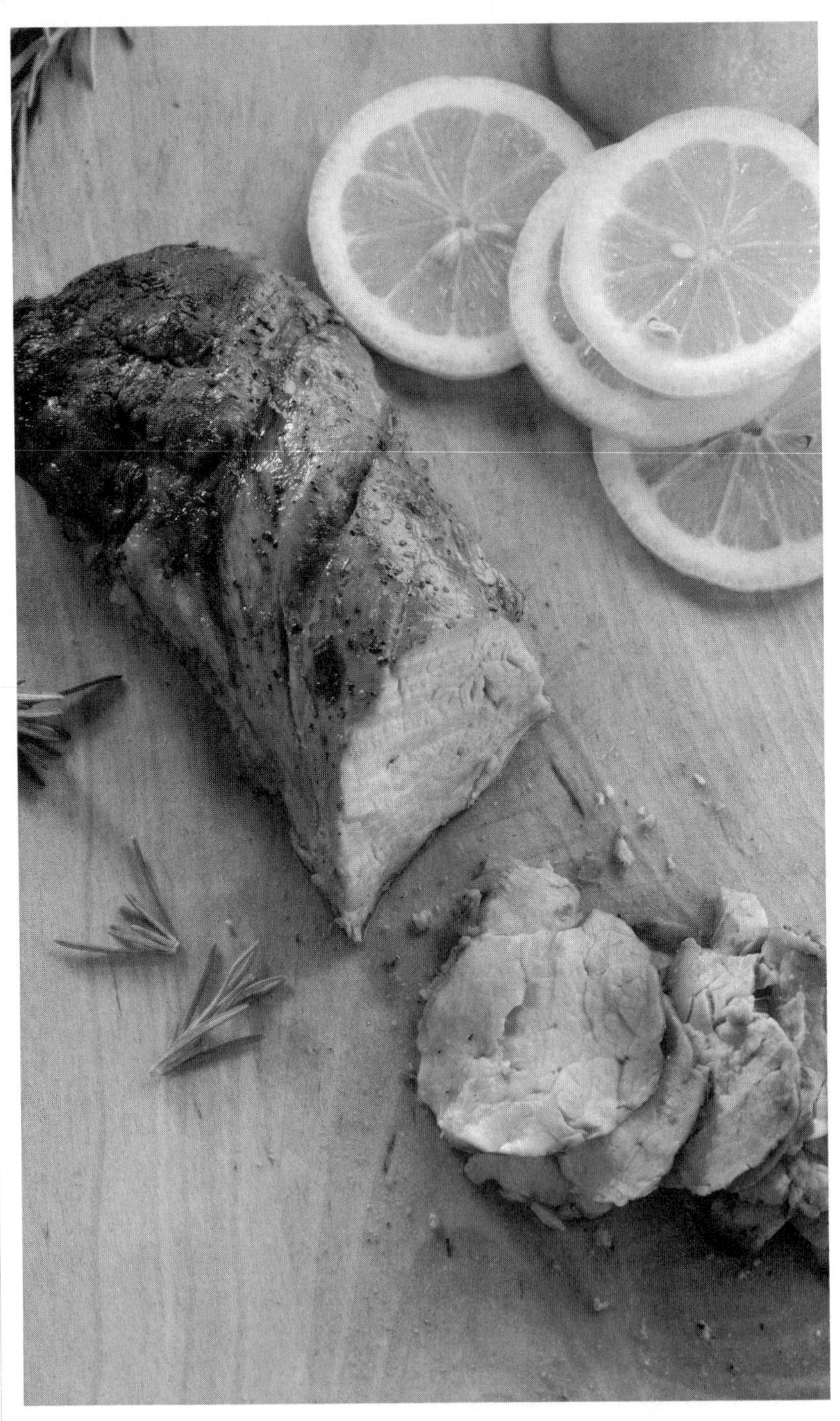

DINNER

- **Lemon and herb pork tenderloin**
- **1 ear, corn on the cob**
- **2 cups mixed greens topped with ½ cup chopped tomato and 2 Tbsp light vinaigrette salad dressing**

Lemon and Herb Pork Tenderloin

SERVES: 4

1 ½ lb pork tenderloin
Juice of one lemon
2 cloves garlic, chopped
1 Tbsp honey
1 Tbsp olive oil
1 Tbsp fresh chopped rosemary
¼ tsp kosher salt
¼ tsp black pepper

1. Place tenderloin in a resealable plastic bag, add lemon juice, garlic, honey, olive oil, rosemary, salt and pepper.
2. Seal and marinate in the refrigerator for one hour.
3. Preheat grill or oven to 400°F.
4. Cook pork for 20 min (5 minutes per side) or until completely cooked through. Allow to rest off the heat for 10 minutes before slicing.

Total Calories: 365 kcal
Total Fat: 11.5 g
Saturated Fat: 3 g
Total Carbohydrate: 27 g
Protein: 40 g
Sodium: 659 mg
Fiber: 5 g

NUTRIENT INTAKE:

29% carbs
43% protein
28% fat

DESSERT

▸ **Peach frozen yogurt (recipe on page 190)**

Calories: 110 kcal
Total Fat: 1 g
Saturated Fat: 0.5 g
Total Carbohydrate: 22 g
Protein: 4 g
Sodium: 33 mg
Fiber: 1 g

NUTRIENT INTAKE:

76% carbs
15% protein
9% fat

NUTRITION FOR THE DAY

Calories: 1358 kcal
Total Fat: 39 g
Saturated Fat: 9.5 g
Total Carbohydrate: 169 g
Protein: 96 g
Sodium: 1831 mg
Fiber: 32 g

NUTRIENT INTAKE:

48% carbs
25% protein
27% fat

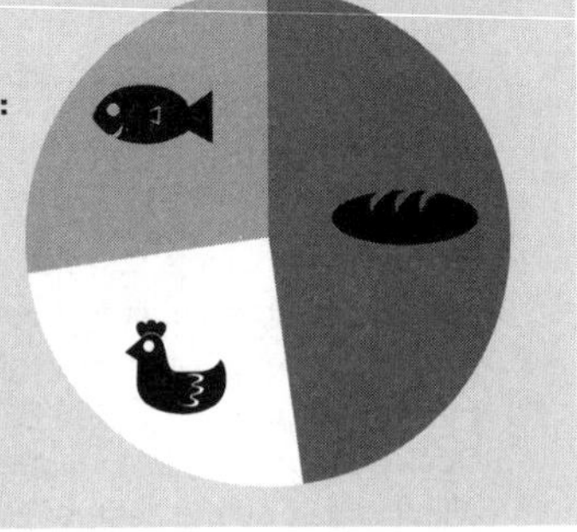

BREAKFAST

- 1 cup cooked steel-cut oatmeal topped with ½ cup sliced strawberries, 2 Tbsp chopped almonds, and 2 tsp maple syrup

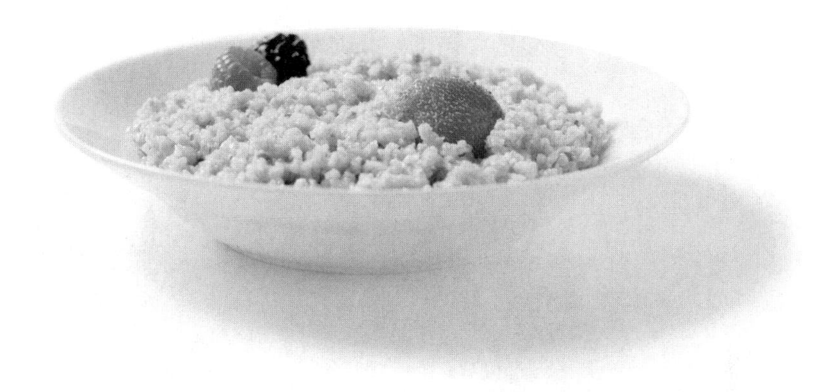

Calories: 283 kcal
Total Fat: 9 g
Saturated Fat: 1 g
Total Carbohydrate: 46 g
Protein: 8 g
Sodium: 2 mg
Fiber: 9 g

NUTRIENT INTAKE:

62% carbs
11% protein
27% fat

SNACK 1

- 10 cherry tomatoes
- ¼ cup hummus

Calories: 134 kcal
Total Fat: 6 g
Saturated Fat: 1 g
Total Carbohydrate: 16 g
Protein: 6 g
Sodium: 245 mg
Fiber: 6 g

NUTRIENT INTAKE:

43% carbs
18% protein
39% fat

LUNCH

▸ **Turkey bacon BLT**

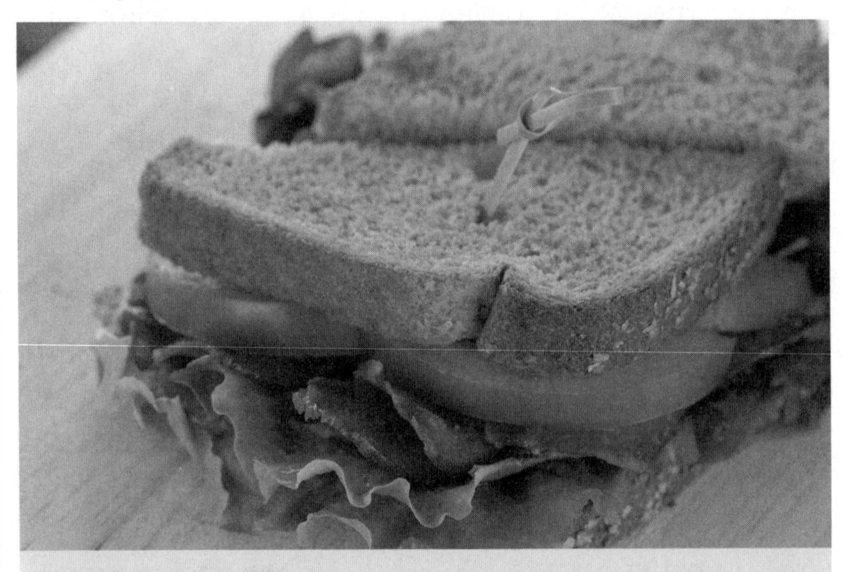

Turkey Bacon BLT

SERVES: 1

2 slices whole wheat bread, toasted
3 slices turkey bacon (3 oz)
3 slices tomato
2 large lettuce leaves

Cook turkey bacon in a nonstick skillet for 3 to 4 minutes per side. Assemble sandwich with turkey bacon, tomato, and lettuce.

Turkey bacon—a MUCH leaner alternative to fatty bacon—works well in just about any recipe that calls for regular bacon.

Calories: 373 kcal
Total Fat: 6 g
Saturated Fat: 2 g
Total Carbohydrate: 44 g
Protein: 35 g
Sodium: 917 mg
Fiber: 7 g

NUTRIENT INTAKE:

47% carbs
38% protein
15% fat

SNACK 2

- **1 medium grapefruit**

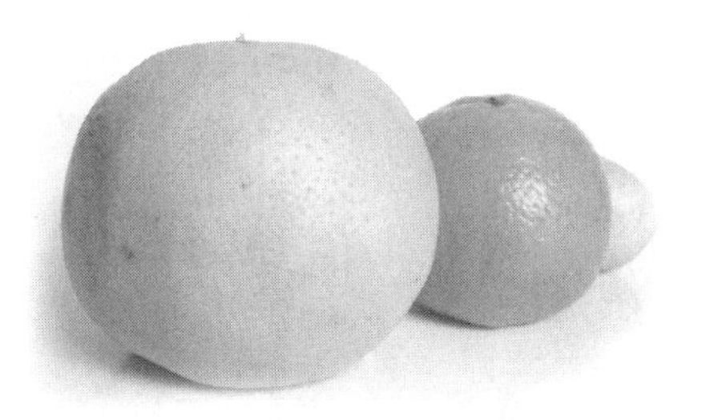

Calories: 82 kcal
Total Fat: 0 g
Saturated Fat: 0 g
Total Carbohydrate: 21 g
Protein: 2 g
Sodium: 0 mg
Fiber: 3 g

NUTRIENT INTAKE:
91% carbs
7% protein
2% fat

SNACK 3

- **10 almonds**
- **1 part-skim mozzarella string cheese**

Calories: 149 kcal
Total Fat: 12 g
Saturated Fat: 4 g
Total Carbohydrate: 3 g
Protein: 10 g
Sodium: 220 mg
Fiber: 1 g

NUTRIENT INTAKE:
8% carbs
24% protein
68% fat

DINNER

- **4 oz grilled salmon**
- **Sautéed zucchini**

Calories: 249 kcal
Total Fat: 10 g
Saturated Fat: 2 g
Total Carbohydrate: 11 g
Protein: 29 g
Sodium: 227 mg
Fiber: 3 g

NUTRIENT INTAKE:
18% carbs
47% protein
35% fat

SNACK 4 (OPTIONAL)

- ½ frozen banana

Calories: 53 kcal
Total Fat: 0 g
Saturated Fat: 0 g
Total Carbohydrate: 13 g
Protein: 1 g
Sodium: 1 mg
Fiber: 2 g

NUTRIENT INTAKE:

93% carbs
4% protein
3% fat

NUTRITION FOR THE DAY

Calories: 1320 kcal
Total Fat: 43 g
Saturated Fat: 10 g
Total Carbohydrate: 153 g
Protein: 90 g
Sodium: 1612 mg
Fiber: 29 g

NUTRIENT INTAKE:

52% carbs
21% protein
27% fat

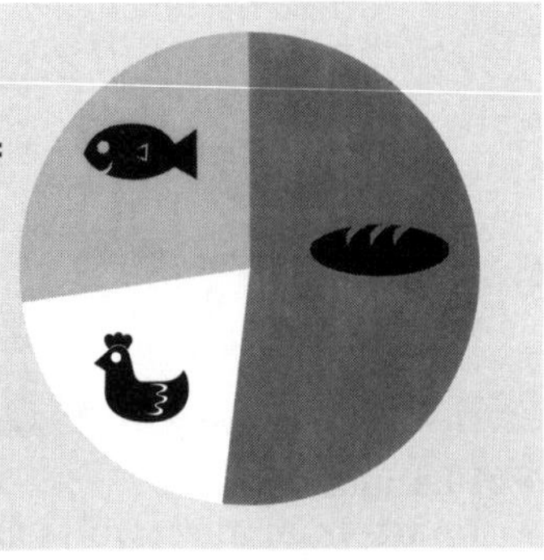

BREAKFAST

- 2 scrambled eggs
- 1 slice whole wheat toast

Calories: 257 kcal
Total Fat: 11 g
Saturated Fat: 3.5 g
Total Carbohydrate: 21 g
Protein: 17 g
Sodium: 290 mg
Fiber: 3 g

NUTRIENT INTAKE:

33% carbs
26% protein
41% fat

SNACK 1

- ½ cup nonfat Greek yogurt
- ¼ cup raspberries

Calories: 76 kcal
Total Fat: 0 g
Saturated Fat: 0 g
Total Carbohydrate: 8 g
Protein: 10 g
Sodium: 43 mg
Fiber: 2 g

NUTRIENT INTAKE:

44% carbs
55% protein
1% fat

LUNCH

- Garden Salad with Chicken

2 cups mixed greens
½ cup sliced cucumber
¼ cup chopped tomato
3 oz grilled chicken breast
¼ cup canned chickpeas, rinsed and drained
2 tsp olive oil
1 Tbsp balsamic vinegar

Calories: 333 kcal
Total Fat: 13 g
Saturated Fat: 2 g
Total Carbohydrate: 23 g
Protein: 31 g
Sodium: 277 mg
Fiber: 6 g

NUTRIENT INTAKE:

28% carbs
38% protein
34% fat

SNACK 2

- **10 almonds**

Calories: 69 kcal
Total Fat: 6 g
Saturated Fat: 0.5 g
Total Carbohydrate: 2 g
Protein: 3 g
Sodium: 0 mg
Fiber: 1 g

NUTRIENT INTAKE:

14% carbs
13% protein
73% fat

SNACK 3

- **1 medium apple**

Calories: 72 kcal
Total Fat: 0 g
Saturated Fat: 0 g
Total Carbohydrate: 19 g
Protein: 0 g
Sodium: 1 mg
Fiber: 3 g

NUTRIENT INTAKE:

96% carbs
3% protein
1% fat

DINNER

- **Spaghetti and meatballs (recipe on page 62)**
- **½ cup sliced cucumber**

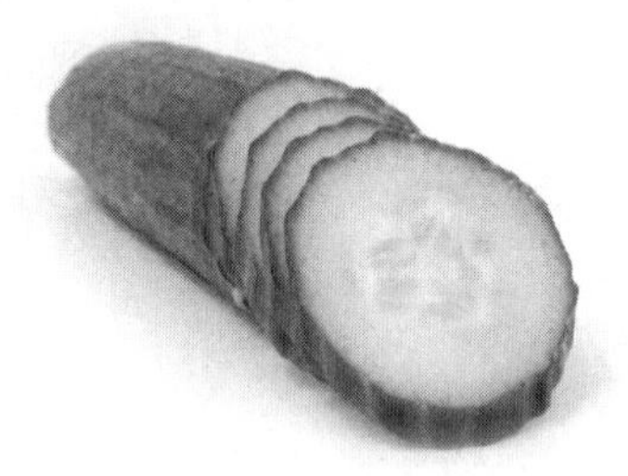

Calories: 480 kcal
Total Fat: 6.5 g
Saturated Fat: 1 g
Total Carbohydrate: 66 g
Protein: 42 g
Sodium: 949 mg
Fiber: 3 g

NUTRIENT INTAKE:

54% carbs
34% protein
12% fat

SNACK 4 (OPTIONAL)

- **1 cup air-popped popcorn**

Calories: 31 kcal
Total Fat: 0 g
Saturated Fat: 0 g
Total Carbohydrate: 6 g
Protein: 1 g
Sodium: 1 mg
Fiber: 1 g

NUTRIENT INTAKE:

77% carbs
13% protein
10% fat

NUTRITION FOR THE DAY

Calories: 1318 kcal
Total Fat: 38 g
Saturated Fat: 7 g
Total Carbohydrate: 146 g
Protein: 104 g
Sodium: 1561 mg
Fiber: 20 g

NUTRIENT INTAKE:

49% carbs
26% protein
25% fat

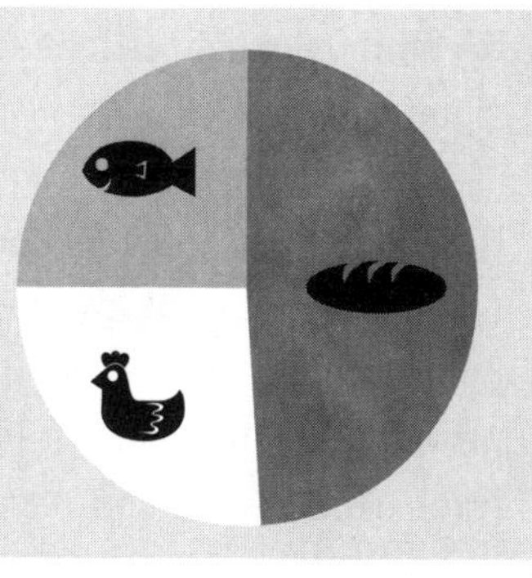

By the end of this meal plan, you should be seeing a significant difference in how you look and feel and in how you approach food and eating. The variety of foods provided in the meal plan were instrumental in helping you achieve Step 1, balancing your daily intake of carbs, protein, and fat. Step 1 helps not only in properly nourishing your body but also in detoxing the body of impurities, allowing the proper conditions for fat burning and weight loss.

The portion sizes for each of the meals were measured with the exact caloric count to satisfy hunger and cravings, reconditioning your mind and body to understand how much food is just enough. This will help you to continue to lose weight as the calories you're taking in have decreased significantly.

Eating frequently throughout the day might have been the hardest step to tackle, but if you've followed through with all the meals, your metabolism should be at an all-time high and burning fat efficiently. Compounded with the perfect balance of nutrients and portion sizes, you've provided an environment for your body to function at its most optimum level. This means you have more energy to be active and get through the day and you're burning fat constantly as you continue to increase your metabolism. As your body continues to work in this efficient way, your waistline will get smaller and unwanted fat will be replaced by lean muscle.

All of these results are just from eating the right foods in the right amounts laid out in the meal plans. Food is powerful at controlling the body, and if used properly, food can change your body for the better and forever.

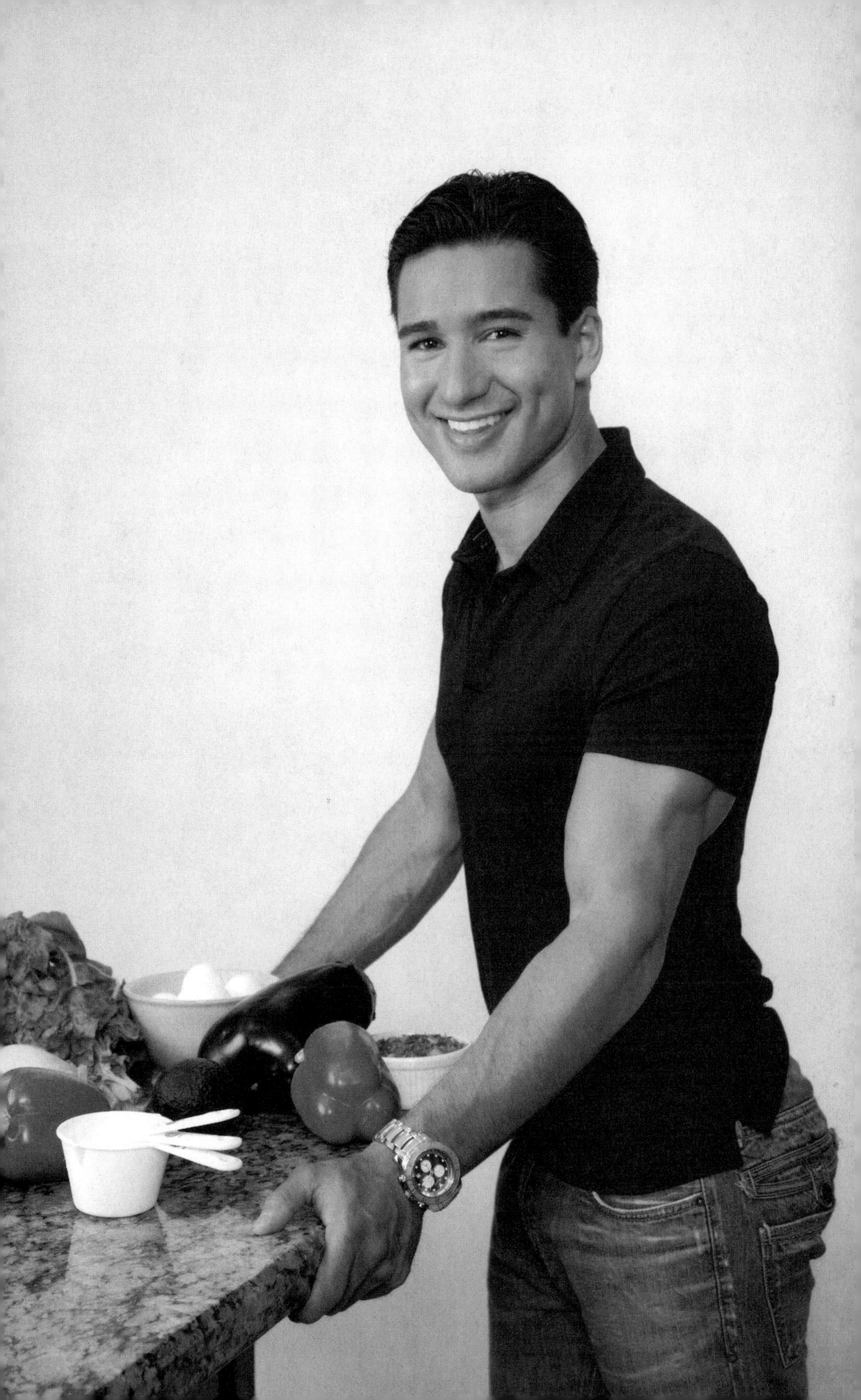

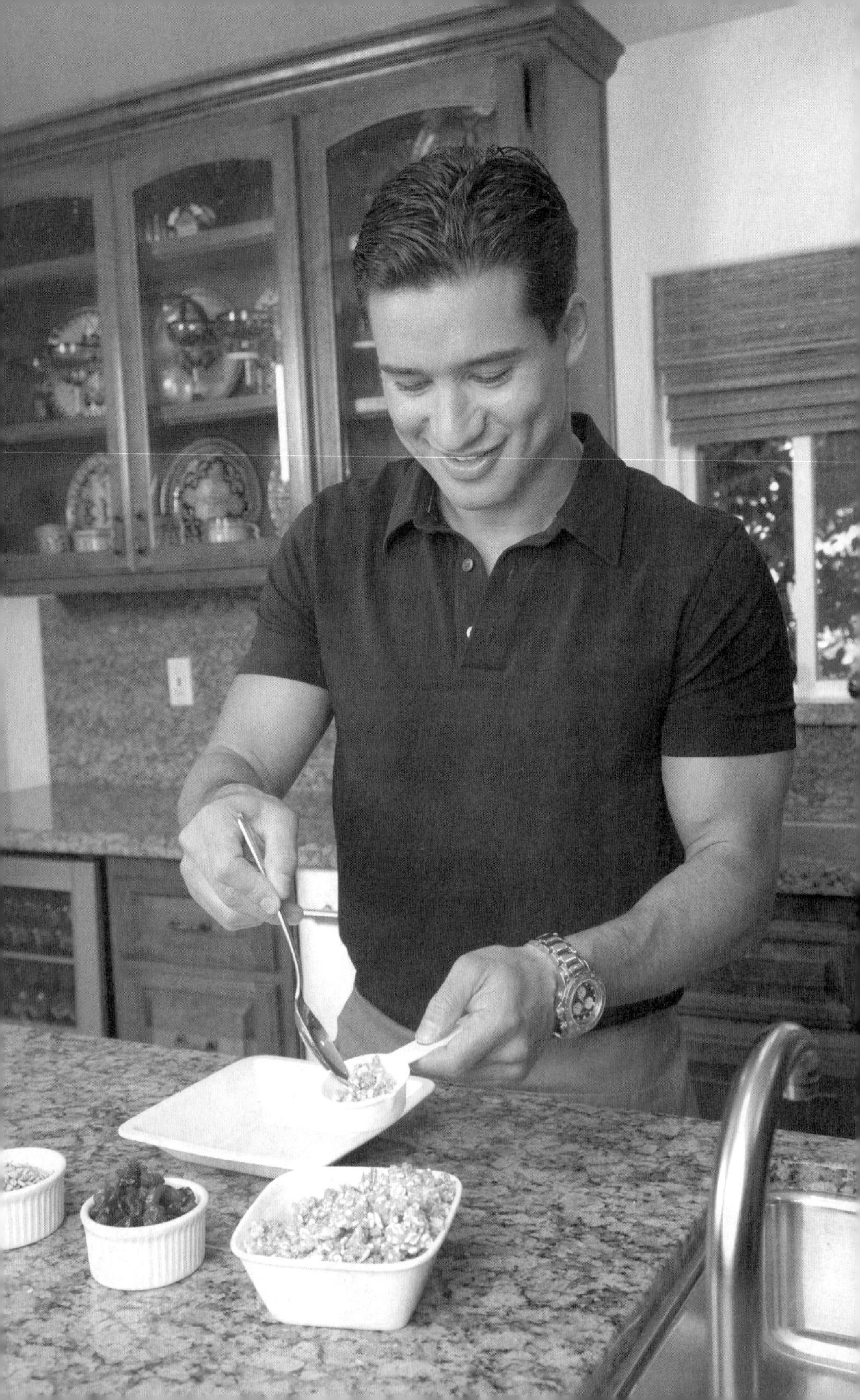

SECTION 3

living extra lean forever

EVEN THOUGH YOU'VE just reached the end of the seven-week meal plan, this is really just the beginning. As I have mentioned constantly, this meal plan was first and foremost designed to teach you how to create the proper conditions for your body to burn fat constantly and efficiently. Once you've learned the extra lean steps and make it your regular routine, your body will continue to unleash the fat-burning properties that will lead to long-lasting weight loss.

Although, there will be times when life gets in the way and it may seem impossible to keep up with the three steps and your new eating habits. The following are a few crucial pointers to tackle those everyday obstacles. Hopefully, these tips will help provide more of the learning and education you need to stay on top of your goals and succeed every day.

living extra lean outside of the home

LIVING EXTRA LEAN is not just limited to healthy eating at home. Granted, it's easier to stick to whole, unprocessed foods when you have prepared and portioned meals and snacks at your disposal. But sometimes life is spontaneous, and you have to learn to roll with the punches. This is where the three steps can really help you to stay on track and make smart choices anywhere you are.

Take for example the other day when I was driving to an interview, but I hadn't eaten in a few hours and I knew I had to fuel up. Well, the only place available to stop on the way was a gas station, and you know how tough it can be to find something healthy at convenience stores. But I was still able to make some good decisions, and fast, since I didn't want to be late for the interview. I ended up finding some low fat, low sodium beef jerky, a banana, and a small bag of unsalted almonds. So right there I found good sources of protein, carbs, and healthy fats, which lasted me a couple of hours through the interview until it was time for another meal. It also goes to show that you can make healthy decisions in the most unlikely places. If you can eat well at a gas station (and you can if you're educated and a little bit clever), you can eat healthy anywhere!

Keep that in mind the next time you're on a road trip and are having a tough time finding a good place to eat.

Here are some handy tips for those times when you are in a pinch and need to refuel fast.

BREAKFASTS

- **1/3 cup Trail Mix**—The healthy combination of dried fruit and nuts will kick-start your metabolism and keep you satisfied until your midmorning snack.
- **Fruit and Nut Bar (LÄRABAR brand recommended)**—This all natural bar made from just fruit, nuts, and spices tastes great and is easy to eat when you're in a hurry.
- **Instant Oatmeal**—Keep packets of instant oatmeal in your desk at work; just add hot water and you've got a breakfast with whole grains and protein that is ready in no time.
- **Yogurt Smoothie**—Bottled yogurt drinks (such as Stonyfield Farm organic yogurt smoothies) are portion controlled, low in fat, and packed with protein and calcium for a quick drinkable breakfast. Choose brands and flavors that are lowest in added sugar.

SNACKS

- **Whole Grains**—Think fiber when you are glancing at that vending machine. Salty or sugary low-fiber foods like chips and cookies will leave you hungry. Look for whole wheat crackers or pretzels when you want something crunchy.
- **Go Nuts**—Healthy fats from nuts are all you need to fight between-meal hunger. Get dry roasted and avoid anything honey roasted, which is coated in oils and extra sugar.
- **Sturdy Fruit**—Bring a few pieces of fruit to work early in the week for daily munching. Choose things like bananas, apples, and oranges that don't require refrigeration and will hold up for the week.
- **Cereal with Nonfat Milk**—Whole grain cereal doesn't have to be strictly breakfast food. A coffee mug full of cereal with some skim milk can be a satisfying snack.

LUNCH AND DINNER

- **Sandwich Stop**—If a quick deli run is your only option, opt for turkey breast, mustard, and any veggies on whole wheat bread. Ask for half the turkey they usually pile on, split with a coworker, or save half for tomorrow's lunch.
- **Low Sodium Soup**—In a pinch, a can of soup makes for a quick microwavable meal. Choose varieties with hunger-fighting fiber and protein like black bean, lentil, or minestrone.
- **Smarter Salad**—Ordering takeout? A garden salad with grilled shrimp or chicken breast is always a safe bet. Ask for vinaigrette dressing on the side and keep portions to 1 or 2 tablespoons.
- **Good Catch**—Broiled or grilled fish like salmon is another healthy take-out option for healthy fat and protein. Ask for it to be prepared without butter and opt for steamed vegetables on the side.

Here are also some smart tips when you find yourself dining out and eating at restaurants:

TIPS FOR EATING OUT/ORDERING TAKEOUT

- Eat prior to going out; trying to "save" calories will lead to overeating
- Look at the menu online ahead of time to avoid impulse ordering
- Avoid fried foods and creamy sauces
- Choose lean meat, fish, whole grains, and vegetables
- Have an appetizer portion as your meal instead of a full-size entrée
- If you drink alcohol, stick to just one drink
- If you have a question about something on the menu (how it's prepared, what it's cooked in), don't be afraid to ask
- Pass on the basket of bread and butter—it's typically empty carbs and unwanted fat
- Get half your dinner to go or share with your spouse or a friend
- Split one dessert with the table instead of eating it alone

SMART CHOICES WHEN DINING OUT

- Miso soup and 2 rolls (12 pieces) of sushi—avoid tempura and creamy sauces and ask for reduced sodium soy sauce
- Veggie or turkey burger with a side salad
- One slice of plain or veggie pizza with a large salad
- Chicken and broccoli (sauce on the side) with steamed brown rice
- Steamed seafood or vegetable dumplings
- Turkey sandwich and fruit salad
- Grilled chicken breast with steamed veggies and a small baked potato
- A bowl of soup (noncreamy) and a salad
- Egg white and veggie omelet with whole wheat toast
- Grilled fish or shrimp with rice and vegetable

answers for permanent weight loss

HERE ARE SOME answers to top frequently asked questions that Dana receives from her clients. One of the most effective ways to stay lean and fit is to constantly educate yourself about food and your body. The more you know about nutrition and how your body responds to food, the more you can be in control.

Is it okay if I drink coffee?

Coffee itself is fine in moderation. It has virtually no calories and actually contains some antioxidants. It's the stuff that you add to coffee that can get you into trouble. The fancy coffee drinks you find at coffee shops nowadays are loaded with unwanted calories from sugar and fat, and adding half-and-half and sugar to regular coffee isn't good either. Some of these drinks you find at Starbucks and other places can have 500 or more calories in them!

So, when you have coffee, stick to low fat or nonfat milk, or better yet, drink your coffee black. And if you want to sweeten it, add a small amount of artificial sweetener instead of sugar. When I go to my local coffee shop, I'm always careful to keep my java as close to black as possible—maybe a little skim milk, but that's it.

As far as caffeine goes, two or three cups of coffee a day (minus the added sugar and fat) is fine. You just want to make sure you don't overdo it, since caffeine is a stimulant. Try not to drink coffee all day long to where by the time your workday is over you've had six or seven cups or more. And certain people will have to be even more careful—people with heart conditions need to be careful with caffeine, and so do pregnant women. So, if you have a preexisting condition, consult your doctor about proper caffeine consumption.

Bottom line, a couple of cups of coffee a day is fine. Just watch what you put into your morning joe!

Is diet soda okay to drink?

The thing about diet soda is that it's generally a better choice than regular soda simply because it doesn't have any sugar. A typical can of regular soda has over 100 calories, and usually closer to 150, depending on the brand. And all of those calories are empty calories from sugar. So, with diet soda, you're saving on calories, but you still want to limit your consumption of it because it contains artificial sweeteners, which are actually chemicals. Artificial sweeteners are safe in small amounts, but you need to be careful with the amount of chemicals you take in through your diet.

It's probably best to limit your intake of diet soda to one or two cans a week. I realize that a lot of people drink much more than that, but that's what I recommend. Outside of sweeteners, some diet sodas are also high in sodium, and others, like colas, have phosphorus in them. Too much phosphorus can actually inhibit your body's ability to absorb calcium, which can be especially harmful for women who have compromised bone health as it is. I know a lot of you like to drink soda (and so do I), but you should really moderate your intake of it, even diet soda.

How about alcohol?

When someone is really serious about losing weight (not to mention living a healthy lifestyle in general), a really good way of keeping calories in check is to avoid alcohol as much as possible. In general, one drink a day for women and two drinks a day for men is what's considered acceptable by medical experts, and there's even research that says that moderate alcohol consumption can actually be good for your health. So if you want to have a drink every now and then, that's fine, but you really have to realize that extra calories are coming along with that alcohol. Take for example the mixed drinks that a lot of restaurants serve, such as margaritas and daiquiris. These drinks in particular are very high in sugar and calories; you could be looking at 500 to 600 calories per drink, and if you have more than one of those, you can see how the calories can add up.

If you're going to have a drink, you're much better off having a small glass of wine or a light beer. Dana has a "100-calorie rule" that she likes to use with her clients to help them remember what's in a drink. Basically, it says that a glass of wine, a light beer, and a shot of alcohol each contain around 100 to 130 calories. So if you have, say, three or four beers or glasses of wine, that can easily amount to over 400 calories. And when Dana says a shot of alcohol has 100 or so calories, that's not counting the mixer you put in it, like soda, orange juice, or tonic water.

I'll be honest, I like to have the occasional drink. My drink of choice is vodka, but I always try to make sure the mixer is something that's calorie free, like seltzer water or diet tonic. You see, even when you're enjoying a drink you can make a smart decision and take advantage of that window of opportunity.

What should I do if I'm going to be out of town for work or vacation? How can I follow the meal plans if I won't be able to prepare my own meals?

In these situations, when cooking your own meals is nearly impossible, just try your best to emulate how the meals are laid out. This is where portion sizes become really important. Hopefully, by the time you go on your trip you've become familiar with some of the meals, which will give you a better feel for how much food you should be eating. By having gone through the meal plans, you'll know how much pasta or rice you should have on your plate or how big the serving of meat should be. I don't expect any of you to bring a measuring cup to a restaurant to figure out how much pasta or rice you should be eating. Eventually, you'll be able to recognize the right amount visually—you'll know what half a cup of rice looks on your plate versus two cups.

So let's say you're in a new city and you're at a restaurant. Look at the meal plan to see what foods it recommends, then try to pick that food either from the menu or by ordering it specially. And you don't always have to choose a meal from the exact week you're on. If you're in Week 5 of the meal plan, it would be great if you could find those exact foods at the restaurant. But if not, feel free to go to another day or week to find something that's similar to what's on the menu.

You might be surprised to find out how easy it is to maintain your healthy eating at a restaurant. If one of the entrées on the menu is a chicken breast smothered in cheese with mashed potatoes on the side, order it without the cheese and with a side of broccoli instead of potatoes. You can always ask your server to have your food prepared differently from the normal way.

Another way to eat healthy when you're traveling is to plan your snacks ahead of time. There are certain snacks you can pack into your luggage very easily. Before you leave home, put a box of healthy granola bars in your bag so that you'll have something to snack on throughout the day. Buy a big bag of almonds and keep those handy. Fix a healthy sandwich and put it in your carry-on so that you have something to eat on a long plane flight. Or, when you arrive in the new city, find a grocery store and stock up on fresh fruit, natural peanut butter, and vegetables. Buy some whole grain cereal and milk and keep it in your hotel room so that you have breakfast taken care of for the entire trip.

The objective is to avoid missing meals when you're traveling and not getting into situations where you're so hungry that you overeat at lunch or dinner. Just because you're traveling doesn't mean you have to get off of your meal plan. All it takes is a little bit of planning ahead of time and, of course, smart decisions when you find yourself at a restaurant or deli.

What should I do when I happen to miss a meal, or miss multiple meals? What's the best way to avoid overeating when I finally do get a chance to eat?

The thing you want to avoid is doubling up, or even tripling up, meals because you miss one or two earlier in the day. In other words, you don't want to give yourself two or three portions of dinner just because you missed lunch and one or both of your afternoon snacks. If you can, have one of the snacks you may have missed an hour or so before you eat dinner, like right after you get home from work and before you start preparing dinner. Even if it's not the normal time you would've had that snack, it can help curb your hunger before dinner, which will make you less likely to overeat. And after dinner, maybe that's a night that you would have the optional snack later on.

The one thing you don't want to do is eat all of your calories for the day (or even most of your calories) at one meal. Dana's meal plans call for 1,200 to 1,400 calories a day, but in order to keep your metabolism high, those calories need to be spread evenly from breakfast to dinner. Having, say, 1,000 calories at dinner means that either you're likely to go over the 1,200 to 1,400 calorie target, or that you've skipped multiple meals prior to that, which has slowed your metabolism and caused you to burn fewer calories.

What if some days I'm not able to eat six to seven times a day? Can I get away with eating four to five times?

Eating four to five times a day is something you can get away with provided you're still meeting your macronutrient and calorie needs (and not exceeding them) over the course of the day. However, in order to maximize your metabolic rate throughout the entire day, eating that fifth and sixth meal, even if they're just small snacks, is more effective. The whole reason I recommend eating six to seven meals a day—not four or five—is that this is the best way to keep you from creating a situation where you're really, really hungry and prone to overeating. If you eat only three or four times a day, at some point you're going to go several hours without eating. This will not only slow your metabolism down, but will also leave you very hungry, which can lead to poor food choices because of such strong cravings.

But I understand that things get busy with work and family and that not every day is a perfect one where you have free time every two or three hours to sneak in a meal. As best as you can, get your six daily meals in, but on those especially hectic days, just make sure you're spacing out those four or five meals evenly and are hitting your daily calorie and macronutrient needs—just as you don't want to exceed those numbers, you also don't want to fall short by eating fewer than 1,200 calories. Not eating enough will catch up to you down the road, usually in the form of overeating.

If I exercise first thing in the morning, should I eat something beforehand or wait until after exercising?

If you can eat something small before you work out, you're probably better off, simply because you want to get your metabolism jump-started as early as possible every morning—basically right after you wake up. Having some food in you can also help give you energy for your workout. At that point, you will have not eaten since the night before (at dinner or your small evening snack), and your body will be ready for some fuel.

Personally, I like to have both protein and carbohydrates before I train, simply because I don't like to work out on an empty stomach, plus I feel like my performance is best if I have both a slow-digesting carb (like oatmeal) and protein in my system. But whatever you decide to eat before working out, just make sure it's something light that you can tolerate and won't cause any discomfort.

But even if you decide to work out on an empty stomach in the morning, it's very important to make sure you don't skip breakfast afterward. I know people who will exercise first thing in the morning on an empty stomach and then go straight to work and oftentimes their first meal isn't until lunch! It might seem like this is a good way to burn calories and lose weight, but it's not. When you skip meals, you slow your metabolism and you're left with lower energy levels; by working out on top of that, you're making the situation even worse—a slower metabolism and even lower energy. You've used all this extra energy at the gym and you haven't replenished any of it. All it takes to keep your body in the right physical state is to make sure you have breakfast right after you exercise.

What role does sleep play in losing weight? Is getting seven or eight hours of sleep going to be better for me than getting four hours?

This is an interesting question, and one that's actually been studied by researchers. It's been shown that sleep-deprived people tend to overeat more than those who get adequate rest. The reasoning behind this is still up in the air, but Dana thinks it could be because being fatigued can lead to decreased willpower, which leads to making poor food choices. From my experiences, I've found that being tired all the time affects my mood and my motivation levels. When I'm chronically tired, I'm not nearly as excited to go to the gym, probably because I'm lacking energy. And when I'm not able to go to the gym on a regular basis, it affects the way I eat. I find that I eat better when I'm hitting the gym hard.

There's also an interesting theory that basically says the more hours you're awake, the more likely you are to want to eat something at times when you don't need food. For example, if you stay up until 3:00 in the morning, chances are you'll be hungry at around midnight, or later, and that's when bad choices can happen—like calling the pizza place that's open all night for delivery! If you're sleeping at 3:00 a.m., however, you won't be thinking about pizza, right?

How do you feel about vitamin and calcium supplements?

Most people, especially women, tend to not get enough calcium in their diets, and even certain vitamins and minerals, so it wouldn't be a bad idea to supplement these. Just a general calcium supplement (even something like Tums will work) and a basic multivitamin are all you would need; you can get the rest of these nutrients from food. In fact, Dana's meal plans were specifically designed to provide sufficient levels of all crucial vitamins and minerals, and even calcium. But different people have different needs. If you have osteoporosis, or even if you just have a family history of it, you may need extra calcium. This is something you can discuss with your doctor.

What you do want to look out for though are products that provide megadoses. According to Dana, with calcium, you don't want to take more than 500 mg at a time. Your body can't absorb any more than that at one time. As for multivitamins, you don't want any supplement that exceeds 100 to 500 percent of your daily recommended value of any vitamin. You'll see some of these multivitamins that have over 1,000% of your daily value of certain vitamins, and you don't need all that.

Is it okay to eat the same thing every day for breakfast or lunch? You talk about how variety is important, but there are a few meals I like much more than others—and they're very healthy meals too!

It's okay to do that every once in a while. Everyone has their favorite foods, and it's okay to eat those foods more frequently than others, but even if those foods are very healthy, you're missing out on whatever nutrients are not in them. So that's where variety becomes very important. Eating the same healthy foods day after day can't take the place of a well-rounded diet, because in a well-rounded diet you're exposing yourself to all the different types of nutrients your body needs as opposed to just focusing on whatever nutrients are in your favorite foods.

My solution to this is: Find new favorite foods! Mix things up and try everything that Dana offers in the seven-week meal plan. By doing that, you'll eat foods you probably never even thought about eating, and there's a good chance you'll discover some new favorites. So when it comes to carbs, don't eat just pasta and potatoes; try quinoa and brown rice. With fruit, don't eat just bananas; eat strawberries, blueberries, pears, and oranges too. With protein, don't stick to just chicken, steak, and eggs; turkey and even pork will provide nutrients those other sources won't. Dana has provided dozens of different recipes, each of which is tasty, healthy, and likely something you've never tried before. She did this so that you can achieve a more well-rounded diet.

Evening and late night snacking is a big problem for me. Do you have any special tips you can suggest for breaking the habit of grazing while I'm at home watching TV at night?

The hope with the meals, and the timing and frequency of these meals, is that you'll satisfy your hunger throughout the day and won't feel the urge to graze at night. This is one of the main reasons Dana selected foods in the meal plans that were nutrient dense, because those are the foods that will satisfy you the most and curb cravings. The main reason people snack constantly at night is because they didn't eat enough during the day and by the time evening rolls around, they're really hungry. I'm hoping this won't be the case once you start following Dana's meal plans.

However, for many people, late night grazing isn't so much a matter of hunger as it is a habit. Whether you've eaten throughout the day or not, you might just have a tendency to want to eat constantly at night, especially when you're watching TV. I think this is more of a psychological tendency; for example, sitting on your couch and watching TV triggers the desire to want to snack on something and have a drink in your hand. This is one reason Dana includes the optional snack a couple of hours after dinner—so that you can feed that craving to some extent.

But that small snack might not be enough to curb your hunger, which is why I've been known to employ a few "tricks" late at night to keep me from driving to the store and buying a box of cookies or a package of M&M'S. The key is to let yourself go through the motions of putting something in your mouth, but to do it with things that don't have calories. Examples include chewing sugarless gum, sipping on herbal tea when you're watching TV (I recommend caffeine-free tea so that it doesn't keep you awake all night), and drinking flavored, noncalorie seltzer water. These kinds of tricks work for a lot of people because they still allow you to keep yourself occupied and not feel like you can't have something to drink while you watch your favorite show. The whole idea is to recognize where your weaknesses are and try to combat them—so if it's cookies, get them out of the house and replace them with high-fiber fruit (apples, pears, oranges) that will make you feel full and keep you from eating more.

Is it okay to eat frozen food, or is that too processed?

With frozen foods, there are two ends of the spectrum. You have things like frozen vegetables and fruit, and then you have frozen entrées. Frozen vegetables and fruit are actually just as healthy as fresh ones, provided they don't have anything added to them like cheese or cream sauce. Plain frozen vegetables have all the same nutrients you'd find in the produce section. Same with frozen fruit—just make sure there's no added sugar in them. Choosing frozen veggies and fruit over fresh can be cheaper (especially when the foods are out of season), not to mention they'll stay good for longer.

On the other hand, prepared frozen foods, even the so-called "healthy" entrées, are heavily processed, have many artificial (and unhealthy) ingredients, and are usually loaded with sodium. These are the types of frozen foods you want to stay away from. These entrées will typically not have the nutrients and fiber you need to stay satisfied and nourished, so do your best to steer clear of these.

Canned tuna is one of my favorite high protein, low carb foods, but I've heard its mercury content is very high. Should I be concerned with that?

Canned tuna is a great protein source and is a good way to get some healthy fish into your diet for those much-needed omega-3 fatty acids. When it comes to mercury, you do want to be careful with some of the fish. For the tuna in the meal plan, there's never more than about a 3- to 5-ounce portion, which is a totally acceptable level. The other fish in the meal plans are low-mercury fish like salmon, cod, tilapia, and so forth.

When choosing a tuna product at the grocery store, *chunk light* tuna is a good choice. People often think "light" means it's lower in calories or fat, but it's not; it's just a different kind of fish, and light tuna tends to be lower in mercury than, say, solid albacore tuna. So if you're concerned with mercury levels, you can certainly choose chunk light over albacore, but if you keep your tuna consumption relatively low (3 to 5 ounces a week) you shouldn't have much to worry about.

What role does sodium play in losing weight and being healthy? How much of it can I get away with?

We all need some sodium in our bodies. Your body uses sodium for a variety of functions, so you definitely need some in your diet. People with high blood pressure need to be careful and might need to cut back on their sodium intake more than those who don't have high blood pressure. But even for healthy individuals, overconsuming sodium can lead to water retention, and no woman (or man, for that matter) likes retaining water, especially when trying to lose weight and look better.

You really want to moderate your sodium intake. The typical recommended amount of sodium is 2,300 mg or fewer per day for someone who doesn't have high blood pressure, so you want to try to stick to that. If you don't eat a lot of takeout and processed foods, 2,300 mg is actually a really easy number to stay below. But when you eat a lot of processed foods, it's not tough at all to blow that number out of the water.

When you're shopping at the grocery store, it's easy find the sodium content of different foods. Just look at the nutrition label on the package—all sodium levels are based on that 2,300 mg amount, so if you see that the daily percentage of sodium in a given food is 50%, or even 100%, you know that's a high sodium food and that you should look for a lower sodium alternative. A quick glance at a food label will go a long way.

When I'm cooking for my family—my kids, of course, aren't following the same meal plans I am—should I cook my meals separately from theirs?

The meal plans weren't designed to be eaten separately from the foods the rest of your family is eating. Remember at the beginning when I talked about the importance of sitting down to the dinner table and enjoying family? This is what it's all about for me, so I would never want you to eat separately from your family!

All the meal plans presented here were designed to be family friendly and can be eaten by anyone—your kids, your husband, your nieces and nephews, whoever. Of course, a teenage boy will likely have different calorie needs from you, so portion sizes will vary. Your fifteen-year-old may be eating more than you, but that doesn't mean you have to cook him a separate meal.

Where the food is concerned, it's wholesome, nutritious, healthy, and also flavorful, which works for anyone. Dana really went out of her way to select foods that everyone, young and old, would like. This is probably my favorite feature of the book—healthy food that tastes great and can be enjoyed by the entire family.

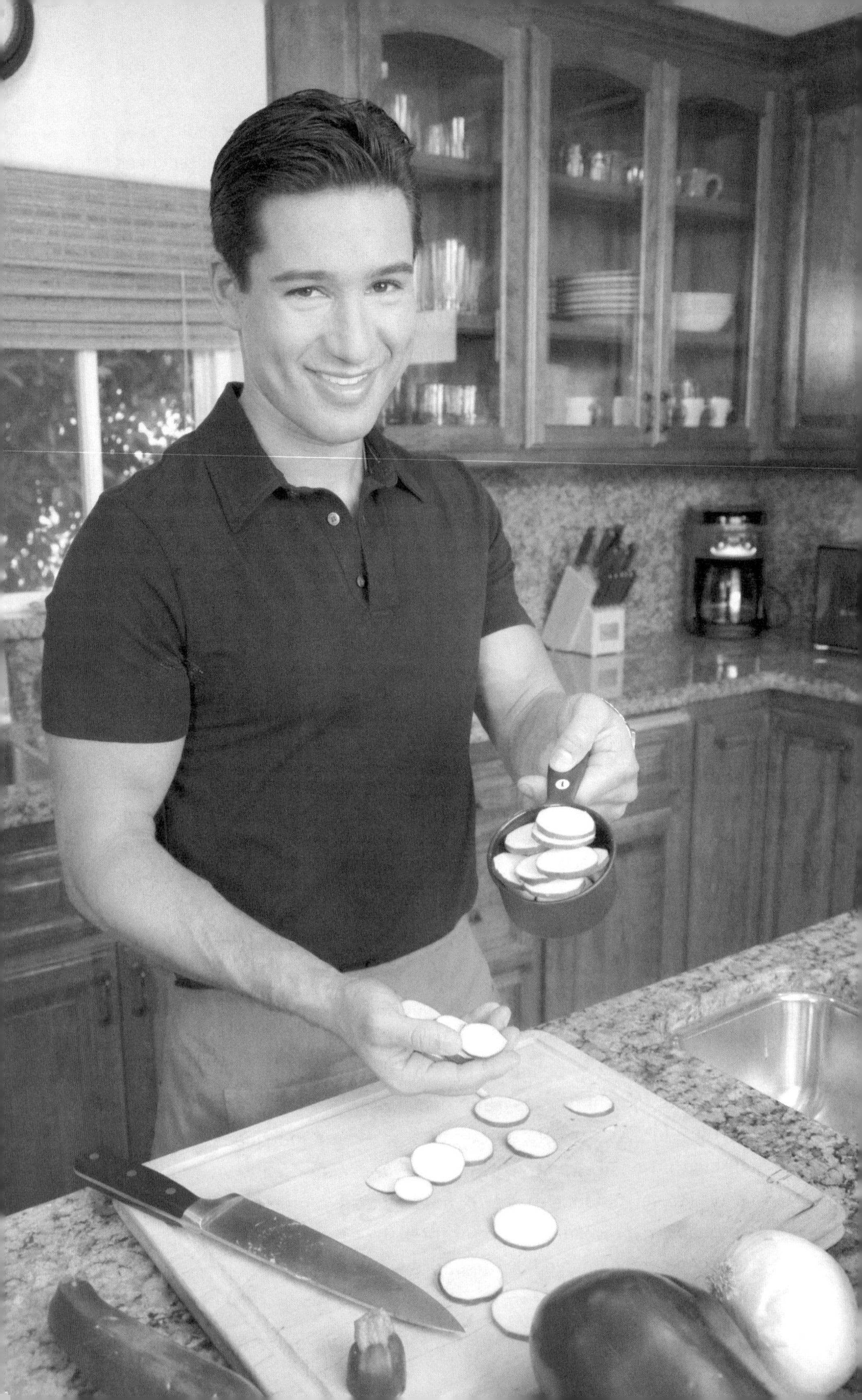

conclusion

SO THIS IS how I eat and this is how I live. If you continue to follow the three steps, you'll be able to naturally maintain your fat-burning body and achieve permanent weight loss for life, while still enjoying food more than ever.

Balance your daily intake of carbs, protein, and fat. Choose a variety of different foods and keep your daily intake to about one-half of carbohydrates, one-quarter of protein, and one-quarter of fat. The right balance of these nutrients prepares your body to create the proper conditions to unleash your natural fat-burning properties, so the first step is a crucial part of weight loss. Don't get stuck in a rut of eating the same foods every day. Likewise, don't adopt some fad diet where protein or carbs take center stage while other important nutrients are put on the back burner. Eat different types of fruits, a wide array of vegetables, stick to lean sources of protein, keep your fiber intake adequate, and don't forget about healthy fats found in fish and nuts.

Practice proper portion control. Simply deciding that you're going to have chicken or a sweet potato at a meal isn't enough; they need to be the right size, neither too big nor too small. The meal plans were specifically designed to teach you what proper portion sizes look like so that you won't have to use a measuring cup or scale for too long. Eating the right portions of food will keep your calorie consumption in check, which is as important as anything when it comes to losing weight.

Eat frequently throughout the day. Keep your metabolism revving high by eating small, frequent meals instead of only one to three large ones every day. The extra lean meal plans call for six or seven meals a day, many of which are small snacks. Overeating at any meal will halt your progress, so stay focused and keep everything in moderation. If it's been a few hours since your last meal, it's time to eat again!

Always enjoy all the food you eat in the right ways that I've taught you in this book. If you make quality food a priority in your life, you are choosing all the benefits of a healthy body: efficient metabolism, nutrient-dense diet, lean body and muscles, increased energy and stamina, and more. Learn to appreciate wholesome food and teach your family and kids to eat fruits and vegetables a little more often and candy and ice cream a little less so. It might seem like a huge and long transition to eat the way that I am asking you to, but remember that controlling the way you eat every day will not only bring you a healthy and lean body, but also liberate you to eat all the foods you want without guilt. Losing weight and changing your eating habits are challenging and difficult in the moment, but remember that you are setting the foundation to enjoy life to the fullest.

Love food. Enjoy life. Live Extra Lean.

Shopping Lists

WEEK ONE Shopping List

▸ Fruits and Vegetables

- ☐ 4 cups chopped tomatoes
- ☐ 1 container cherry tomatoes
- ☐ 2 apples
- ☐ 3 bananas
- ☐ 3 oranges
- ☐ 1 red onion
- ☐ 1 bag grapes
- ☐ orange juice
- ☐ 2 plums or tangerines
- ☐ 1 small carton of strawberries
- ☐ 3 cups diced red bell pepper
- ☐ 2 sweet potatoes
- ☐ 4 heads of broccoli
- ☐ 2½ cups spinach
- ☐ 1 bag of celery
- ☐ 2 limes
- ☐ 1 zucchini
- ☐ 1 bag of baby carrots
- ☐ 1 bag of mixed greens
- ☐ ¼ cup of black olives
- ☐ 3 cucumbers
- ☐ 3 cloves garlic
- ☐ dried or fresh parsley
- ☐ 1 ginger root
- ☐ 1 cup hummus
- ☐ fresh basil
- ☐ almonds
- ☐ slivered almonds
- ☐ sunflower seeds
- ☐ box of raisins

▸ Cheese/Dairy

- ☐ 4 Tbsp. low fat feta
- ☐ 4½ cups nonfat vanilla yogurt
- ☐ 1 bag of 2-part-skim mozzarella string cheese
- ☐ 1 cup Greek yogurt
- ☐ 1 bag of frozen mixed berries
- ☐ skim milk
- ☐ sugar-free chocolate pudding

▸ Meats, Seafood, and Eggs

- ☐ 10 oz. grilled chicken breast
- ☐ 1½ lbs ground turkey breast
- ☐ 4 oz. flank steak
- ☐ 4 oz. salmon
- ☐ 12 oz. low sodium turkey
- ☐ 4 oz. cooked shrimp
- ☐ dozen eggs

▸ Canned

- ☐ 1 can black beans
- ☐ 1 can tomato paste
- ☐ 28-oz. can diced tomatoes

▸ Grains/Pastas

- ☐ oatmeal
- ☐ brown rice
- ☐ whole wheat English muffins
- ☐ small container of seasoned bread crumbs
- ☐ 1 whole wheat tortilla
- ☐ loaf of whole wheat bread
- ☐ 1 cup whole grain cereal
- ☐ 8 oz. whole grain pasta (Barilla a plus)
- ☐ natural peanut butter
- ☐ 2 granola bars (Kashi: 130 calories)

▸ Spices

- ☐ salt and pepper
- ☐ teriyaki or horseradish sauce
- ☐ reduced-sodium soy sauce
- ☐ Dijon mustard
- ☐ cumin
- ☐ chili powder
- ☐ canola oil
- ☐ dried oregano
- ☐ white wine vinegar
- ☐ extra-virgin olive oil
- ☐ cinnamon
- ☐ honey
- ☐ light vinaigrette dressing
- ☐ barbecue sauce

WEEK TWO Shopping List

▸ Fruits and Vegetables

- ☐ container of blueberries
- ☐ 3 pears
- ☐ 1 tomato
- ☐ grape tomatoes
- ☐ grapefruit
- ☐ chopped pineapple
- ☐ cantaloupe
- ☐ ¼ cup unsweetened applesauce
- ☐ 4 carrots
- ☐ large bag of baby carrots
- ☐ bag/container of shelled edamame
- ☐ broccoli
- ☐ green beans
- ☐ 1 cucumber
- ☐ 1 eggplant
- ☐ 2 red onions
- ☐ cauliflower
- ☐ large bag of mixed greens
- ☐ 2 tangerines
- ☐ 4 red bell peppers
- ☐ 1 small baked potato
- ☐ bag of green peas
- ☐ 1 head or bag of lettuce
- ☐ walnut halves
- ☐ slivered almonds
- ☐ popcorn
- ☐ dried cranberries
- ☐ sunflower seeds
- ☐ box of raisins

▸ Cheese/Dairy

- ☐ nonfat cottage cheese
- ☐ nonfat vanilla frozen yogurt
- ☐ skim mozzarella string cheese
- ☐ low fat buttermilk
- ☐ skim milk
- ☐ grated Parmesan cheese
- ☐ nonfat plain yogurt

▸ Meats, Seafood, and Eggs

- ☐ sliced chicken breast lunch meat
- ☐ 3 grilled chicken breasts
- ☐ grilled shrimp
- ☐ 4 oz. wild salmon
- ☐ 4 oz. flank steak
- ☐ 6 oz. canned tuna
- ☐ 4-oz. pork chop
- ☐ 2- to 2½-lb turkey breast (bone in, skin on)
- ☐ 4 eggs
- ☐ 2 egg whites

▸ Canned

- ☐ 2 small containers of sugar-free gelatin
- ☐ 1½ cups Amy's low sodium lentil soup
- ☐ ¼ cup canned chickpeas
- ☐ 1 can black beans
- ☐ 1 can tomato paste
- ☐ 1¾ cups low sodium chicken or vegetable broth
- ☐ small container of tomato paste
- ☐ natural peanut butter

▸ Grains/Pastas

- ☐ 2 cups oatmeal
- ☐ 2 pitas
- ☐ 2 Kashi granola bars
- ☐ whole wheat bread
- ☐ 1¼ cups whole grain cereal
- ☐ 1¼ cups all-purpose flour
- ☐ 1½ cups quinoa
- ☐ 6 whole wheat crackers

▸ Spices

- ☐ 1 bottle honey
- ☐ 1 bottle olive oil
- ☐ 1 bottle extra-virgin olive oil
- ☐ maple syrup
- ☐ cinnamon
- ☐ sugar
- ☐ salt
- ☐ black pepper
- ☐ 1 head garlic
- ☐ 4 cloves garlic
- ☐ canola oil
- ☐ Dijon mustard
- ☐ 2 tsp. fresh thyme
- ☐ light vinaigrette salad dressing
- ☐ reduced-sodium soy sauce
- ☐ teriyaki or hoisin sauce
- ☐ ginger root
- ☐ grill seasoning
- ☐ lemon juice
- ☐ 1 lemon (enough to get ½ tsp. lemon zest)
- ☐ vanilla extract
- ☐ balsamic vinegar
- ☐ baking powder

WEEK THREE Shopping List

▸ Fruits and Vegetables

- ☐ 3 bananas
- ☐ 3 mangoes
- ☐ 4 apples
- ☐ frozen pineapple chunks
- ☐ 3 containers of raspberries
- ☐ pineapple
- ☐ 4 tomatos
- ☐ celery
- ☐ Swiss chard
- ☐ butternut squash
- ☐ romaine lettuce
- ☐ 2 large bags of mixed greens
- ☐ sweet potato
- ☐ small jar of black olives
- ☐ scallions
- ☐ small bag of frozen corn kernels
- ☐ 3 cucumbers
- ☐ zucchini
- ☐ 2 red onions
- ☐ red bell pepper
- ☐ large bag of arugula
- ☐ jalapeño pepper (optional)
- ☐ dried apricots
- ☐ orange juice
- ☐ 20 celery stalks
- ☐ cashews
- ☐ popcorn

▸ Cheese/Dairy

- ☐ 1 cup nonfat plain Greek yogurt
- ☐ 3 slices low fat Swiss cheese
- ☐ 3 part-skim mozzarella string cheese
- ☐ skim milk
- ☐ 1 oz. dark chocolate

▸ Meats, Seafood, and Eggs

- ☐ 8 oz. low sodium roast beef
- ☐ 15 oz. grilled chicken breast
- ☐ 3 oz. grilled turkey breast
- ☐ 4-oz. pork chop
- ☐ 5 oz. salmon
- ☐ 8 oz. shrimp
- ☐ 4 eggs
- ☐ 2 egg whites

▸ Canned

- ☐ vegetable broth
- ☐ 2 28-oz. cans crushed tomatoes
- ☐ 15-oz. can tomato sauce
- ☐ 15-oz. can garbanzo beans
- ☐ 15-oz. can red kidney beans
- ☐ 15-oz. can black beans

▸ Canned (*cont.*)

- ☐ almond butter
- ☐ 1½ cups Amy's lentil soup or black bean soup (low sodium)
- ☐ 1 small container of sugar-free gelatin (optional)
- ☐ canned chickpeas
- ☐ nonstick cooking spray

▸ Grains/Pastas

- ☐ oatmeal
- ☐ toasted wheat germ
- ☐ tortilla chips
- ☐ 2 6-inch whole wheat tortilla
- ☐ frozen whole grain waffles
- ☐ whole grain cereal
- ☐ 2 slices whole wheat bread
- ☐ 1¼ cups whole wheat couscous
- ☐ whole wheat pasta

▸ Spices

- ☐ salt and pepper
- ☐ caesar dressing
- ☐ olive oil
- ☐ kosher salt
- ☐ 1 clove garlic
- ☐ ground cumin
- ☐ Worcestershire sauce
- ☐ 1 cup dark beer
- ☐ cayenne pepper
- ☐ 2 Tbsp. chili powder
- ☐ celery salt
- ☐ dried tarragon
- ☐ Dijon mustard
- ☐ grill seasoning
- ☐ lemon juice
- ☐ lime juice
- ☐ canola oil
- ☐ reduced-sodium soy sauce
- ☐ honey
- ☐ light vinaigrette
- ☐ fresh basil
- ☐ teriyaki sauce
- ☐ balsamic vinegar

WEEK FOUR Shopping List

▸ Fruits and Vegetables

- ☐ 2 containers of blueberries
- ☐ 2 containers of strawberries
- ☐ 3 pears
- ☐ 5 oranges
- ☐ orange juice
- ☐ cranberry juice cocktail (optional)
- ☐ 3 medium containers of cherry tomatoes
- ☐ 1 cucumber
- ☐ small bag of frozen corn
- ☐ 3 heads of broccoli
- ☐ baby spinach
- ☐ arugula
- ☐ spinach
- ☐ 2 heads or packages of lettuce
- ☐ 1 bell pepper
- ☐ 3 avocados
- ☐ 1 package of extra-firm tofu
- ☐ green cabbage
- ☐ 1 carrot
- ☐ 2 medium sweet potatoes
- ☐ 1 large bag of mixed greens
- ☐ 1 onion
- ☐ almonds

▸ Cheese/Dairy

- ☐ 2 containers of nonfat Greek yogurt
- ☐ low fat cheddar cheese
- ☐ skim milk
- ☐ 2 6-oz. containers of nonfat fruit or vanilla yogurt
- ☐ unsalted butter

▸ Meats, Seafood, and Eggs

- ☐ cooked chicken (enough for 1 cup diced chicken)
- ☐ 12 oz. grilled chicken breast
- ☐ frozen grilled chicken sausage
- ☐ 1 lb. ground turkey breast
- ☐ 4 oz. broiled flank steak
- ☐ 4 oz. salmon
- ☐ 5 oz. tilapia
- ☐ 6 eggs
- ☐ 2 egg whites

▸ Canned

- ☐ sun-dried tomatoes (packed in oil)
- ☐ 1½ cups canned chickpeas
- ☐ olives
- ☐ container of hummus
- ☐ 4 oz. canned tuna
- ☐ nonstick cooking spray
- ☐ salsa

▸ Grains/Pastas

- ☐ steel-cut oatmeal
- ☐ 1 Tbsp. toasted wheat germ
- ☐ bulgur wheat
- ☐ 4 brown rice cakes
- ☐ whole wheat English muffin
- ☐ granola bars (Kashi: 130 calories)
- ☐ cornstarch
- ☐ whole grain cereal
- ☐ whole wheat tortilla
- ☐ 2 large graham crackers (optional)
- ☐ 2 slices whole wheat bread
- ☐ 2 frozen whole grain waffles
- ☐ flour
- ☐ rolled oats
- ☐ brown rice (small package)

▸ Spices

- ☐ salt and pepper
- ☐ kosher salt
- ☐ black pepper
- ☐ 4 lemons (some to be used for lemon zest)
- ☐ 2 limes
- ☐ olive oil
- ☐ lemon juice
- ☐ parsley
- ☐ cilantro (optional)
- ☐ dark sesame oil
- ☐ reduced-sodium soy sauce
- ☐ rice vinegar
- ☐ hoisin sauce
- ☐ canola oil
- ☐ ginger root
- ☐ light vinaigrette salad dressing
- ☐ maple syrup
- ☐ 2 tsp. light mayonnaise
- ☐ natural peanut butter
- ☐ natural fruit spread
- ☐ sugar
- ☐ light brown sugar

WEEK FIVE Shopping List

► Fruits and Vegetables

- ☐ 2 containers of strawberries
- ☐ 1½ cups diced watermelon
- ☐ 2 bags of grapes
- ☐ 1 orange or 2 tangerines
- ☐ 2 tangerines or plums (optional)
- ☐ 1 tangerine
- ☐ 2 containers of applesauce
- ☐ 3 apples
- ☐ 3 bananas
- ☐ 3 tomatoes
- ☐ green beans
- ☐ Swiss chard
- ☐ 1 container of shelled edamame
- ☐ 1 large bag of mixed greens
- ☐ small container of celery
- ☐ 1 small bag of spinach
- ☐ 1 bag of baby spinach
- ☐ arugula
- ☐ 3 red bell peppers
- ☐ 2 cucumbers
- ☐ eggplant
- ☐ mushroom
- ☐ 3 red onions
- ☐ 1 medium sweet potato
- ☐ 1 container of walnuts
- ☐ 1 container of almonds
- ☐ sunflower seeds
- ☐ popcorn
- ☐ dried cranberries

► Cheese/Dairy

- ☐ 1 container of nonfat cottage cheese
- ☐ 3 part-skim mozzarella string cheese
- ☐ Parmesan or Pecorino Romano cheese
- ☐ cheddar cheese
- ☐ skim milk
- ☐ 1% milk
- ☐ reduced-fat cream cheese
- ☐ Swiss cheese
- ☐ unsalted butter
- ☐ 1 oz. dark chocolate

► Meats, Seafood, and Eggs

- ☐ 15 oz. chicken breast
- ☐ 9 oz. low sodium turkey breast
- ☐ 4 oz. pork tenderloin
- ☐ 5 oz. grilled fish (such as mahi-mahi or cod)
- ☐ 7 egg whites
- ☐ 2 eggs

▸ Canned

- ☐ 5 oz. canned tuna
- ☐ 1½ cups Amy's black bean soup or lentil soup
- ☐ natural peanut butter
- ☐ natural fruit spread
- ☐ 1 can low sodium vegetable broth or chicken broth
- ☐ tomato paste
- ☐ nonstick cooking spray

▸ Grains/Pastas

- ☐ 2 whole wheat English muffins
- ☐ 1 6-inch whole wheat pita
- ☐ 2 small bags of whole wheat pretzels
- ☐ 4 slices whole wheat bread
- ☐ whole grain cereal
- ☐ quinoa
- ☐ cooked oatmeal
- ☐ 1 lb. whole grain elbow macaroni
- ☐ flour

▸ Spices

- ☐ salt
- ☐ Dijon mustard
- ☐ black pepper
- ☐ kosher salt
- ☐ low fat vinaigrette salad dressing
- ☐ olive oil
- ☐ extra-virgin olive oil
- ☐ 3 cloves garlic
- ☐ fresh thyme
- ☐ balsamic vinegar
- ☐ lemon juice
- ☐ mayonnaise
- ☐ honey
- ☐ white wine vinegar
- ☐ Worcestershire sauce
- ☐ ground nutmeg
- ☐ red peppers
- ☐ dried oregano
- ☐ barbecue sauce

WEEK SIX Shopping List

▸ Fruits and Vegetables

- ☐ frozen mixed berries
- ☐ chopped pineapple (enough for 3 cups)
- ☐ orange juice
- ☐ 4 peaches
- ☐ 3 oranges
- ☐ container of raisins
- ☐ 2 containers of blueberries
- ☐ 2 tomatoes
- ☐ large container of cherry tomatoes
- ☐ container of grape tomatoes
- ☐ onion
- ☐ large bag of mixed greens
- ☐ 1 head or bag of romaine lettuce
- ☐ 1 head or bag of lettuce
- ☐ 4 heads of broccoli
- ☐ 2 cucumbers
- ☐ green beans
- ☐ celery strips
- ☐ 2 red onions
- ☐ bell pepper
- ☐ mushrooms
- ☐ baby spinach
- ☐ 1 carrot
- ☐ frozen green peas
- ☐ lemon
- ☐ 3 sweet potatoes
- ☐ package of extra-firm tofu
- ☐ cashews

▸ Cheese/Dairy

- ☐ 1 container of nonfat vanilla yogurt
- ☐ 5 containers of nonfat fruit yogurt or vanilla yogurt
- ☐ container of nonfat Greek yogurt
- ☐ low fat Swiss cheese
- ☐ Parmesan cheese
- ☐ low fat shredded cheese
- ☐ low fat feta cheese
- ☐ skim milk
- ☐ 2 cups of sugar-free, fat-free chocolate pudding
- ☐ low fat buttermilk

▸ Meats, Seafood, and Eggs

- ☐ 11 oz. chicken breast
- ☐ 9 oz. low sodium roast beef
- ☐ 4 slices of low sodium roast beef
- ☐ 4 oz. pork tenderloin
- ☐ 4 oz. wild salmon
- ☐ 3 oz. raw shrimp
- ☐ 6 eggs

▶ Canned

- ☐ 3 oz. canned tuna
- ☐ 4 oz. turkey breast
- ☐ almond butter
- ☐ chickpeas
- ☐ nonstick cooking spray
- ☐ anchovy paste

▶ Grains/Pastas

- ☐ 2 granola bars (Kashi: 130 calories)
- ☐ 1 slice whole wheat bread
- ☐ 1 6-inch whole wheat tortilla
- ☐ 1 whole wheat tortilla
- ☐ 3 brown rice cakes (2 are optional)
- ☐ whole grain cereal
- ☐ 2 whole wheat English muffins
- ☐ whole wheat couscous
- ☐ whole wheat flour
- ☐ flour

▶ Spices

- ☐ salt
- ☐ black pepper
- ☐ Dijon mustard
- ☐ olive oil
- ☐ extra-virgin olive oil
- ☐ lemon juice
- ☐ Worcestershire sauce
- ☐ minced garlic
- ☐ mayonnaise
- ☐ light vinaigrette dressing
- ☐ low fat vinaigrette
- ☐ balsamic vinegar
- ☐ sesame oil
- ☐ fresh parsley
- ☐ honey
- ☐ canola oil
- ☐ 1 clove garlic
- ☐ salsa
- ☐ sugar
- ☐ baking soda
- ☐ vanilla extract
- ☐ maple syrup
- ☐ baking powder

WEEK SEVEN Shopping List

▸ Fruits and Vegetables

- ☐ 2 containers of strawberries
- ☐ 1 large container of raspberries
- ☐ 3 pears
- ☐ 3 apples
- ☐ 5 peaches
- ☐ 3 grapefruits (1 optional)
- ☐ 2 bananas
- ☐ 2 heads of broccoli
- ☐ cabbage
- ☐ celery
- ☐ 1 large head or bag of lettuce
- ☐ 2 bell peppers
- ☐ 2 tomatoes
- ☐ 2 large bags of mixed greens
- ☐ 1 ear of corn
- ☐ container of cherry tomatoes
- ☐ 2 zucchinis
- ☐ large bag of baby carrots
- ☐ carrots
- ☐ 2 avocados
- ☐ 1 cucumber
- ☐ lime (for lime juice)
- ☐ lemon (for lemon juice)
- ☐ hummus
- ☐ 2 onions
- ☐ almonds
- ☐ popcorn
- ☐ package of extra-firm tofu

▸ Cheese/Dairy

- ☐ 4 part-skim mozzarella string cheese
- ☐ Parmesan cheese
- ☐ 1 cup plain low fat yogurt
- ☐ 1 cup plain low fat Greek yogurt
- ☐ 2 cups nonfat Greek yogurt
- ☐ skim milk

▸ Meats, Seafood, and Eggs

- ☐ 16 oz. chicken breast
- ☐ grilled chicken sausage
- ☐ 4 oz. low sodium turkey breast
- ☐ turkey bacon
- ☐ 1 lb. ground turkey breast
- ☐ 1½ lb. pork tenderloin
- ☐ 4 oz. grilled flank steak
- ☐ 4 oz. grilled salmon
- ☐ 5 eggs
- ☐ 2 egg whites

▸ Canned

- ☐ natural peanut butter
- ☐ 1½ cups of Amy's low-sodium lentil soup or black bean soup
- ☐ canned tuna
- ☐ chickpeas
- ☐ tomato paste
- ☐ 28-oz. can diced tomatoes

▸ Grains/Pastas

- ☐ steel-cut oatmeal
- ☐ brown rice
- ☐ 4 slices whole wheat bread
- ☐ whole wheat crackers
- ☐ whole wheat couscous
- ☐ cornstarch
- ☐ whole grain cereal
- ☐ whole wheat tortilla
- ☐ seasoned bread crumbs
- ☐ 8 oz. whole grain pasta

▸ Spices

- ☐ salt
- ☐ kosher salt
- ☐ black pepper
- ☐ maple syrup
- ☐ salsa
- ☐ olive oil
- ☐ 6 cloves garlic
- ☐ dried or fresh oregano
- ☐ red pepper flakes
- ☐ sugar
- ☐ balsamic vinegar
- ☐ light vinaigrette salad dressing
- ☐ fresh cilantro (optional)
- ☐ mayonnaise
- ☐ honey
- ☐ sesame oil
- ☐ reduced-sodium soy sauce
- ☐ rice vinegar
- ☐ hoisin sauce
- ☐ canola oil
- ☐ ginger root
- ☐ rosemary
- ☐ fresh basil

Acknowledgments

THERE ARE MANY people to thank, but let me single out the following individuals whose help and support was truly immeasurable:

My publisher, Ray Garcia, my editor Kim Suarez and the entire team at Penguin. When your vision collided with your dedication, my dream came true. 1,000 times, thank you.

My manager, Mark Schulman, for climbing the tallest trees in my career, allowing me to always head in the right direction. Nice call on this one.

My writer, Jimmy Peña, and his team, Joe Wuebben and Dana Angelo White, for your tireless contributions to this project.

Mom, Marissa and the rest of my family of chefs. Thank you for teaching me the joy of family and food. What's for dinner?

index

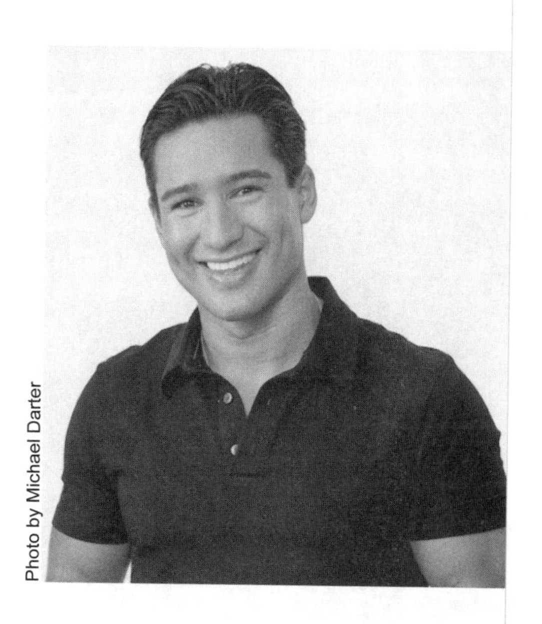
Photo by Michael Darter

MARIO LOPEZ is currently the host of TV's second-longest-running entertainment show, *Extra*, and MTV's highest-rated program, *Randy Jackson Presents America's Best Dance Crew*. He is also the author of the children's book *Mud Tacos* and the workout book *Knockout Fitness*.